Dublin, 1745–1922

THE MAKING OF DUBLIN CITY

Series Editors
Joseph Brady and Anngret Simms
Department of Geography
University College Dublin

Joseph Brady and Anngret Simms (eds), *Dublin through space and time, c.900–1900*

Ruth McManus, *Dublin, 1910–1940: shaping the city and suburbs*

Niamh Moore, *Reinventing Dublin's docklands* (forthcoming)

Gary A. Boyd, *Dublin, 1745–1922: hospitals, spectacle and vice*

Joseph Brady, *Living in the city, 1940–2000: a social and economic geography* (forthcoming)

Dublin, 1745–1922

HOSPITALS, SPECTACLE AND VICE

Gary A. Boyd

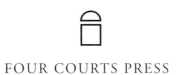

FOUR COURTS PRESS

Set in 11 pt on 14 pt Garamond by
Carrigboy Typesetting Services, County Cork for
FOUR COURTS PRESS LTD
7 Malpas Street, Dublin 8, Ireland
e-mail: info@four-courts-press.ie
http://www.four-courts-press.ie
and in North America for
FOUR COURTS PRESS
c/o ISBS, 920 NE 58th Avenue, Suite 300, Portland, OR 97213.

© Gary A. Boyd and the editors 2006

ISBN 1–85182–960–1 hbk
ISBN 1–85182–966–0 pbk

All rights reserved. No part of this publication may be
reproduced, stored in or introduced into a retrieval system,
or transmitted, in any form or by any means (electronic, mechanical,
photocopying, recording or otherwise), without the prior
written permission of both the copyright owner and
publisher of this book.

Printed in England
by MPG Books, Bodmin, Cornwall.

Contents

7
ACKNOWLEDGMENTS

9
SERIES EDITORS' INTRODUCTION

11
INTRODUCTION

13
LABOUR IN A LANDSCAPE OF PLEASURE

A new hospital for Dublin – Landscapes of hospitality: Dublin hospitals in the eighteenth century – Founding hospitals – Hospital practice in the eighteenth century – Male-midwifery and the founding of the Dublin Lying-in Hospital – The form of the first Lying-in Hospital – The controversies of a maternity hospital – Mosse's first use of theatre – The colonial landscape – Kildare House: rural harmony in the city – Kildare House and the new Lying-in Hospital: a comparison – Landscapes of pleasure – The separated spheres of labour and leisure – Protestantism and productivity

75
THE HOSPITAL AND THE SPECTACULAR CITY

The death of Mosse – The arrival of Charlemont and the Rotunda – Utility and ornament – Colonizing the landscape of care: other hospitals in mid-eighteenth-century Dublin – The Knights of St Patrick and the Assembly Rooms – The emergence of Rutland Square – The Wide Streets Commissioners – A city divided: the limits of the Wide Streets Commissioners' interventions

123
DUBLIN AND ITS DEMI-MONDE

Sex and the pleasure garden – The clients and memoirs of Mrs Leeson, madame – Ambiguities and contradictions at the Lying-in Hospital –

Tension and desire in the Lying-in Hospital chapel – The Magdalen Asylum and the Bethseda chapel – Vice and the closure of the Pleasure Gardens

144
SPACES OF EMPIRE

A militarized society – Prostitution, venereal disease and the Westmoreland Lock Hospital, Dublin – The Hospital for Incurables – From house to machine: Richard Johnston and the Westmoreland Lock Hospital – Disease, morality and further extensions at the Lock Hospital – Moral management at the Lock Hospital – Visibility and order: other institutions by Francis Johnston – The creation of Monto – Statisticians, morality and public space – Monto: labyrinth of vice?

194
EPILOGUE
The city as theatre – Backstage Dublin

202
APPENDIX

207
BIBLIOGRAPHY

217
LIST OF ILLUSTRATIONS

220
INDEX

Acknowledgments

In order to complete this work I received a great deal of help and advice and I owe a great deal of thanks. Firstly, I would like to thank the series editors: Dr Joseph Brady for his technical expertise in the production of the volume and Professor Anngret Simms for her invaluable and tireless editorial work. This book developed from my doctoral thesis which was undertaken at the School of Architecture, University College Dublin, and benefited enormously from the counsel and knowledge of my supervisor, Dr John Olley. The critical insights of my colleagues Dr Hugh Campbell and Dr Finola O'Kane were also both encouraging and influential as was the input of the external examiners of my thesis, professors Adrian Forty (University College London) and Murray Fraser (University of Westminster). Doctor Yvonne Whelan deserves thanks for her advice and support in the initial stages of transforming my thesis into a book. I thank Professor Loughlin Kealy and all the staff and students at the School of Architecture for their continuing support. Special thanks must go to Paul Kenny, Pierre Jolivet and Gerry Hayden. I would also like to thank the Master and staff at the Rotunda Maternity Hospital, especially Ray Philpott, for allowing me access to the building. Thanks also to the staff at the Royal College of Physicians, especially to the librarian Robert Mills, who allowed me unlimited use of the Westmoreland Lock Hospital records. In equal measure, I would like to express my appreciation of the many people in various archives and respositories who helped me, particularly those in the National Archives; the Dublin City and County Libraries, the Irish Architectural Archive; the National Library; Kilmainham Gaol Archives, and the Special Collections of University College Dublin. Very special thanks are due to Julia Barrett, Sheila Astbury and all in the School of Architecture Library. The final preparation of the book for the publishers was undertaken in the Department of Geography, University College Dublin and I owe much to the skill of Stephanie Halpin and Stephen Hannon.

Credit must also be given to friends who have suffered, almost as much as I have, the mood swings, the pleasures and frustrations of writing a book. They know who they are. Finally I would like to pay thanks to two families. My mother and late father who have always been and always will be inspirational figures in my life, as is my grandmother, whose support and open-mindedness has always encouraged me and Blair, for his brotherly advice. I must also thank the Hanley family, especially Hugh and Josephine but most of all, of course, my wife Anna, without whom none of this would have been possible.

Series editors' introduction

Some years ago we embarked on a series of books entitled *The Making of Dublin City* with the aim of bringing knowledge of the growth and development of the city to a wide audience in a manner that would be both scholarly and entertaining. As geographers, we were particularly concerned to put forward a view of the city from our perspective, where the focus was on the streetscape and the forces and processes that have shaped it and continue to shape it. Visual imagery was particularly important in telling our story and the books are noteworthy for the number of illustrations they contain. The first volume in the series, *Dublin through space and time*, looked at significant episodes in the growth of the city from its origins as a small Viking trading base to the beginnings of the twentieth century when it stood on the brink of its enormous suburban expansion. This suburban expansion was the focus of the second volume, *Dublin, 1910–1940*, in which Ruth McManus looked at the early suburban housing schemes and the complex relationships between public and private sectors. Further volumes are in preparation that will continue the story of the growth of the city to the present day.

We always intended that we would produce thematic volumes that would explore some aspect of the city in more detail. This volume is the first such book and it will soon be joined by a book on the development of Dublin's docklands.

Dublin in the eighteenth century became famed for the elegance of its streets and its architecture, particularly the developments of the Wide Streets Commission. It is often forgotten that the centre of Dublin at the time of the Act of Union was seen by many international commentators as a jewel of European planning. The wealth and opulence that this landscape suggested was, of course, shared only by a relatively small group of people and there was a significant underbelly to the city where the realities of daily life were far removed from the world of promenade and sedan chairs. On a leisurely walk down eighteenth-century Sackville Street (now O'Connell Street) you would have encountered well-dressed ladies and gentlemen, who enjoyed being seen and wanted to be admired. But, in Malton's prints of that time you also see men in rags courageously confronting elegant men on horseback to beg for a few coins or women huddled with babies in their arms in street-corners waiting to receive small gifts of money. The nineteenth century was less kind to the city to the degree that Dublin became famed for its beggars and degradation rather than its landscapes.

Dr Gary A. Boyd of the School of Architecture, University College Dublin, explores the contradictions between the visual landscape and the social realties of the city in the eighteenth century by looking at a nether world that few of us would have imagined. He brings to life the people recorded in the archives of the Rotunda Hospital, the Lock (venereal) Hospital and the Hospital of Incurables. These hospitals played a very important, but often veiled, role in maintaining public health in the city and assisting those on the very edge of society at a time when social services as we would know them were unknown. The book gives a fascinating account how the Rotunda, the world's first maternity hospital built at the far end of elegant Sackville Street, fitted into the social and political fabric of the city of that time. The New Pleasure Gardens, on the site of to-day's Parnell's Square, were ostensibly built to provide funds for the new hospital, but they also introduced new types of social engagement and entertainment to the city, which focused on spectacle and display. The establishment of the Hospital of Incurables and the Lock Hospital are interpreted by Gary A. Boyd as attempts by the ruling élite to purify urban spaces and remove disturbing sights from public gaze. This arose out of a sense of civil and religious responsibility in an effort to keep up the appearances of an ideal Protestant city. There is, therefore, a constant tension in the city between public positions and private life that is reflected in the manner in which the city is used.

Architects and geographers have a great deal in common in how they view and understand the world around them and Gary A. Boyd is very much at home in this series. The author takes us by the hand and shows us how space and architectural forms combined to produce spaces with new meanings. We see how the lower classes in their desperate physical needs were accommodated into this new urban landscape and architectural framework. Through his account we see, with new eyes, a landscape that we believed we understood.

JOSEPH BRADY & ANNGRET SIMMS

Introduction

This book began life as an investigation into the relationship in contemporary Dublin between, what seemed to me, to be its official city of monuments, museums, galleries, shops and civic areas and an unofficial city, the *terra incognita* of alleyways, vacated buildings, empty lots and other marginalized or leftover spaces. Space in the first city seemed highly controlled and designed to facilitate only a limited band of formal and prescribed activities and accordingly, many of the activities which did not fit in were often accommodated in the more secluded realm of back stage Dublin. A few months after the research began, however, I was confronted with a revelation which changed the course and scope of the investigation. In an interview with a police officer involved in the operation of the Closed Circuit Television (CCTV) camera network in the Temple Bar area of the city, he disclosed that in any such systems there are inevitable 'shadows'. These are places where, due to the positioning of the cameras on a pre-existing landscape, the urban topography of twisting streets, undulations and the presence of trees or other plantings, obstruct the facility's scope of vision. More strikingly, however, was that the existence and indeed, the geometry of these zones were well known to certain sections of Dublin's criminal fraternity. To illustrate this point, the policeman pointed to a small triangular area on the map of Temple Bar whose 'shading' from the CCTV cameras had apparently contributed to it being the locus of a miniature crime wave. Even in one of the most tightly controlled public areas of the city, therefore, certain uncontrollable and unpredictable activities existed.

My attention at this point turned to the architectural histories of well-known public spaces and buildings in Dublin which I was in the process of reading as background context. If unofficial types of activity could still flourish under the intense pressure of twentieth-century surveillance technology, then surely historic public spaces must have been home to a lively gamut of activities and phenomena which sat outside the expected and prescribed, or even the legal or moral. The histories, however, were on the whole strangely reticent. On the rare occasions when they did discuss the relationship between architectural space and the activities it accommodated, it was only briefly and on the most obvious of terms, focusing firmly on those activities which are automatically invoked by a building's title or category – hospital, chapel, prison, church, post office, etc. Moreover, when describing a building's form, detail and decoration, any deviation from an accepted series of rules of style was generally considered an aberration with no further significance.

Convinced that these, for the most part well-renowned and well-discussed spaces, were the sites of more complex patterns of human interaction and undiscovered connections between space, form, decoration and behaviour, I set a course for the *terra incognita* of Dublin's architectural history and began to explore the gaps left in its traditional accounts. This, of course, does not mean such accounts are not of value, but merely that it is necessary to extend their scope of investigation to provide alternative means of interpreting and understanding space. Often, the presence of hidden complexities in a building's life is strikingly evident within those very idiosyncratic elements in its form or function which seem to disrupt the rules of architectural or, indeed, social convention. Accordingly, we begin in mid eighteenth-century Dublin, at the apparently bizarre juxtaposition of a maternity hospital and a 'leisure centre'.

Labour in a landscape of pleasure

A new hospital for Dublin

At 9 a.m. on 4 June 1751, a group of dignitaries including the lord mayor left the tholsel in the centre of Dublin, crossed the river Liffey and proceeded in state to the New Pleasure Gardens in Great Britain Street (now Parnell Street) on the northern edge of the city. There, Bartholomew Mosse (Figure 1), founder of the Lying-in Hospital, looked on as the foundation stone for the institution's next development, a new, purpose-built hospital, was laid on this the birthday of the prince of Wales (later George III) by the lord mayor. Not everything, however, was as it seemed. At the ceremony, Mosse admitted, in a whispered aside to a colleague, that he was only worth five hundred pounds, whereas the new hospital would take twenty thousand to build. His solution to these financial irregularities showed a finely gauged understanding of the uses of spectacle. Mosse gave the lord mayor and his retinue a splendid breakfast followed by 'genteel and liberal entertainments', an act of largesse which made it seem as if he was a person of substantial means (Wilde, 1846, p. 573).

In fact, the gesture was curiously appropriate to the site. As their name implied, the New Pleasure Gardens – opened by Mosse in 1748 to provide funds for the hospital – constituted a landscape dedicated to the production of pleasure and spectacle. Boasting the newest and most exotic, magnificent and fantastic entertainments in the city, the gardens rapidly assumed a privileged position in the social web of Dublin's leisured classes. And when the new hospital finally opened in 1757, it added another layer to the gardens' already burgeoning list of exquisite attractions – a magnificent backdrop, constructed in the latest Palladian style of architecture. By the 1770s, not only was the area famous as one of Dublin's most fashionable resorts, it had also acquired some of the city's most exclusive private addresses.

All this, however, represented a stark contrast to the circumstances of the hospital's original establishment at George's Lane, south east of the castle in the city's squalid old town, only twelve years earlier in 1745 (Figure 2). There, amidst humble and insalubrious surroundings, Mosse had created in a domestic outhouse the first maternity hospital in the British Isles. The hospital's transformation in fortunes can be partly attributed to the persuasive abilities of Mosse, who, as the unlikely, but apparently charismatic persona of

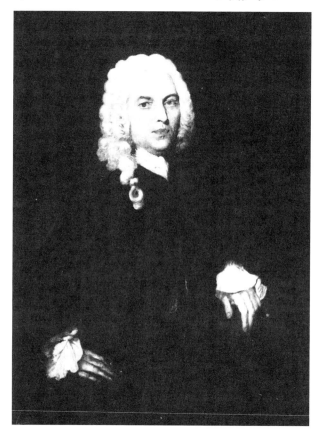

1 Bartholomew Mosse. (Unknown, c.1745, in the possession of the Rotunda Hospital.)

a surgeon, man midwife and entertainment impresario, managed to woo and ultimately convince a set of aristocratic sponsors unrivalled by any other charitable institution in the city, to support a hospital dedicated to the practice of male midwifery, an unfashionable and often controversial pursuit.

Mosse's personal charisma, however, was only one of a number of factors which influenced the development of Dublin's maternity hospital. Dublin, in common with other British cities, gradually accumulated a whole series of new hospitals over the course of the eighteenth century. The majority of these were so-called 'voluntary hospitals' – institutions which were funded privately and owed their continuing existence and future expansion to the benevolence of sponsors and patrons. And while the rising number and larger sizes of these hospitals over the course of the century could be seen as a necessary consequence of the exponential population and urban growth of cities, the reality was more complex.

It has been suggested, for example, that, among its other purposes, the frequently magnificent architecture of the eighteenth-century hospital on mainland Britain (and elsewhere in Europe) often served as a vehicle for the celebration and self-aggrandisement of its sponsors and patrons (Stevenson, 2000; Foucault, 1991, 1993). In eighteenth-century Ireland, however, the rise

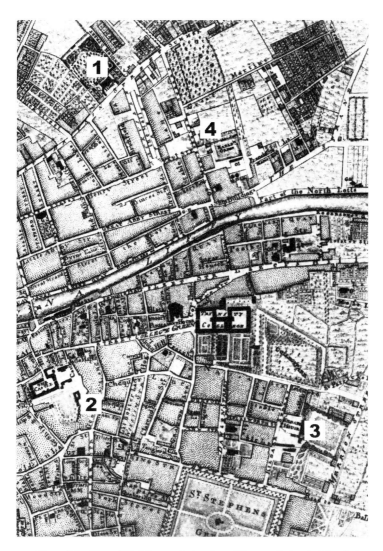

2 Plan of the City of Dublin, 1756, showing **1** The new Lying-in Hospital (opened 1757) and gardens; **2**: its original site at George's Lane, south east of the castle (opened 1745); **3** Kildare House; **4** Tyrone House. (John Rocque, Plan of the City of Dublin, 1756, with author's numbers added.)

of the voluntary hospital took place in a colonial context with its sponsors generally being representatives of the powerful, yet often insecure, Protestant Anglo-Irish settler class. In such circumstances, the production of an architecture of self-edification perhaps acquires an additional potency. Indeed, when set against a uniquely sparse Irish institutional landscape – the combined results of the dissolution of the monasteries in the sixteenth century and the subsequent non-extension of the Elizabethan poor law of 1601 to Ireland – the provision of care and the development of the hospital had the potential to be more immediately ideologically or politically charged than elsewhere. This is perhaps intensified in the idea of a maternity hospital. In an island which was being extensively remade not only in the colonizer's image, but also under a new, capitalistic re-organization of agriculture, the arrival of an institution so strikingly dedicated to issues of productivity assumes a deeper significance. Similarly, the New Pleasure Gardens, with its new opportunities for leisure, can be thought of as part of a rapidly widening sphere of consumption.

Meanwhile Mosse, as well as deriving his social position from a family heritage closely associated with colonial intervention, was also a representative of the socially aspirant professional class. In Mosse's case, however, his chosen profession of obstetrics was fraught with insecurities and, for much of the eighteenth century, was involved in a struggle to achieve recognition and acceptance. Dublin's Lying-in Hospital and pleasure gardens, therefore, represented the intersection of many diverse but interconnected cultural, social and personal landscapes. These, once embodied in space, would have profound implications for the subsequent development of both the social life and urban form of Dublin city.

Landscapes of hospitality: Dublin hospitals in the eighteenth century

In the early 1740s, Dublin possessed four recently established voluntary hospitals: the Charitable Infirmary (1718), Steeven's Hospital (1733), Mercer's Hospital (1734), and the Hospital for Incurables (1743). In addition, there were three older institutions located around the edges of the city which were also known as hospitals, but whose function was slightly different: the Hospital of King Charles or Bluecoat School (begun in 1671), the Royal Hospital Kilmainham (begun in 1680) and the Foundling Hospital (created in 1729 in, and as part of the Poor House, 1703; Figure 3). The differences between the newer and older examples provide an opportunity to clarify what

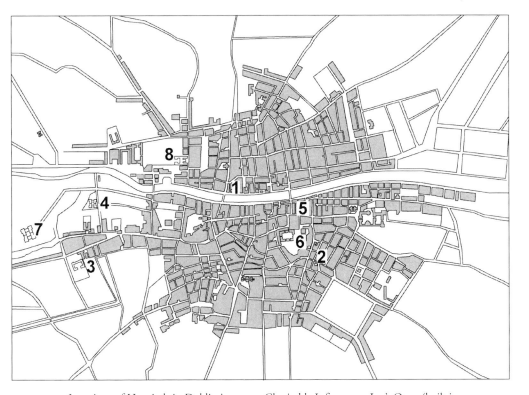

3 Locations of Hospitals in Dublin in 1745: **1** Charitable Infirmary – Inn's Quay (built in 1730 and rebuilt on the same site in 1741, previously on Cook Street, founded in 1718); **2** Mercer's Hospital (founded 1727, opened 1734); **3** Foundling Hospital (founded 1729, as part of the Poor House which was originally built in 1703); **4** Steeven's Hospital (founded 1733); **5** Hospital for Incurables – Blind Quay (founded 1743); **6** Lying-in Hospital – George's Lane (founded 1745); **7** Royal Hospital, Kilmainham (begun 1680); **8** Bluecoat Hospital (begun 1671). (Compiled by the author, based on John Rocque, *Exact Survey*, 1756.)

the concept of hospital actually meant in the eighteenth century. The words hospital, hospice, hostel and hotel are all derived from the Latin *hospes*, meaning the guest of the host. They reflect the variety of functions of the medieval hospital as: hospital, almshouse, asylum, orphanage, foundling home, guest-house for travellers and pilgrims, poor-house etc. (Pevsner, 1976, p. 193).

The medieval or *ancien régime* hospital, then, was not necessarily concerned with the curing of its visitors or inhabitants, but rather afforded a wide range of services from basic necessities like food and accommodation to rudimentary forms of care. These hospitals, moreover, were frequently founded and operated with an overtly religious ethos, administering as much to the spiritual needs of the patients and the prospects of their souls in the afterlife, as to their bodily needs in the present one. However, as implied above, the word hospital also often had a more secular context as a 'house of hospitality' – a type of inn or even a manor house. Throughout the eighteenth century, the older meanings of hospital lingered on stubbornly during the slow process of what has subsequently been termed 'medicalization'. The path towards a medical hospital began with a break from an inclusive and undifferentiating acceptance of almost all those seeking admission – where sickness was only one among a range of factors, including infirmity, old age, inability to find work etc. – to a more distinguishing policy of admitting only those who stood a reasonable chance of being cured by the application of medical and surgical methods. Thus, the meaning of hospital gradually began to shift to become associated with a productive process – with an end product of a healthy and useful citizen – rather than simply a container for social misfits or the sick poor's penultimate destination (Foucault, 1991, p. 276).

In Dublin, the Royal Hospital Kilmainham (essentially a retirement home for ex-soldiers), the Foundling Hospital (a type of orphanage), and the Blue-Coat hospital (a place for the sustenance and relief of poor children as well as 'aged and impotent people'), broadly represented the older type of hospital, whose inhabitants' condition was social and therefore lay beyond the limits of what medicine could reasonably achieve. The purported differences between these institutions and the new, voluntary hospitals are perhaps best exemplified by the notices which appeared throughout the eighteenth century in publications such as Watson's *Gentleman and Citizen's Almanack*. These contained statistics related to admissions, but perhaps more significantly, the number of patients at the new hospitals who had been 'discharged as cured'. To begin with, the modest scale of Dublin's first voluntary hospitals also distinguished them from the 'ceremonious but inept architecture' (Foucault, 1991, p. 278) of the older institutions moored to the city's edges (Figures 4, 5, 6 and 7). However, as the following notice for Mercer's Charitable Infirmary illustrates, ambiguities still remained between notionally scientific 'physical and surgical advice' and a concern for the bodily comfort and hospitality associated with the older type:

> A great number of such poor sick, maimed or wounded Persons, as appear to be curable and proper Objects are there relieved. Physical and surgical advice and medicines are given to all. Sixty-five sick Poor have at one time been supplied with Diet, Washing, Lodging and Medicines within the House.
>
> (Watson's *Almanack*, 1750)

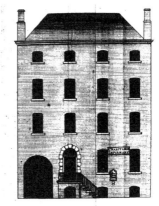
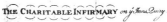

4 The Charitable Infirmary on Inn's Quay, 1730. (*Dublin Magazine*, 1763.)

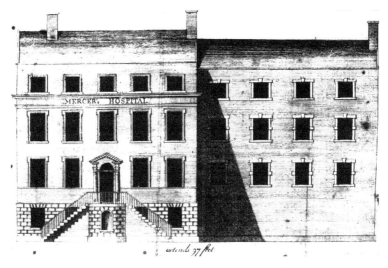

5 Mercer's Hospital, founded 1727, extended 1757. (Engraving after J. Aheron, 1762.)

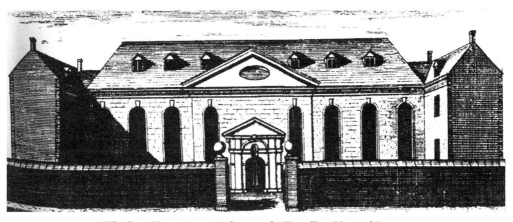

6 The Poor House in 1728; it became the Foundling Hospital in 1729. (Charles Brooking, 1728.)

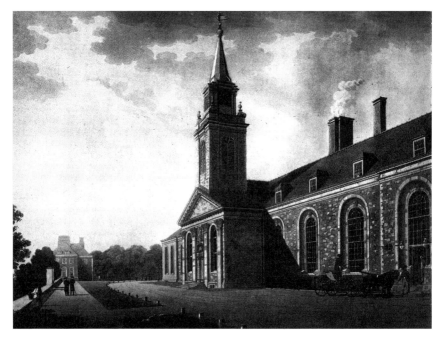

7 The Royal Hospital, Kilmainham. (James Malton, 1799.)

As the break between the older and newer hospital types was not always entirely clear, the modern voluntary hospital often found itself the recipient of some of the same criticism which had beset its predecessors. The vast, decrepit and often squalid medieval Hôtel Dieu in Paris, for example, was often described in the eighteenth century as an 'ante-chamber to death' – an insalubrious place from which patients were unlikely to return. Despite its purported modernizing principles, the voluntary hospital struggled, not only with this negative legacy but also, at a time when it was not yet entirely distinct from the poor-house, to justify its very existence as a separate institution (Stevenson, 2000 p. 8).

Founding hospitals

Most of the voluntary hospitals in Dublin were founded by surgeons and, with a few exceptions, almost all of these were in humble domestic premises. The conversion of a house to a hospital was relatively straightforward. Essentially unburdened by ideas of contagion or ventilation, or the necessity of differentiated spaces, the process often simply involved fitting out the rooms in a house with as many beds as physically possible. Most hospitals, however, were remarkably small by today's standards: the Charitable Infirmary, for example, founded in Cook Street in 1718, had only four beds. Moreover, almost all of the Dublin hospitals which began life in appropriated domestic property, were located within the narrow and confined precincts of the older, medieval part of the city. Some of these original sites were reused by different hospitals at different times. For example, the Lock Hospital (for venereal patients), one of the city's most peripatetic, occupied the vacated building of the original Lying-in Hospital in George's Lane after the latter moved to its new site in 1757. In fact, in their early years many hospitals had a relatively nomadic existence and the apparent ease with which they could relocate from site to site in the city seems to reiterate their non-specific spatial requirements.

The use of domestic premises, however, tended to represent an intermediary stage towards purpose-built hospitals. Purpose-built often also meant *larger* and was usually accompanied by a relocation from the congested old centre to sites farther out in newer suburbs or on the city's edges. The Charitable Infirmary, for example, moved from Cook Street to Jervis Street; the Lock Hospital, from George's Lane to Townsend Street; and the Meath Hospital, from the Coombe to Long Lane on the city's southern periphery. There were, however, notable exceptions. St Catherine's, St Nicholas', the Dublin and the Charitable Venereal Hospitals, for example, had only ephemeral existences and, having failed to secure new premises, disappeared after only a few years. Steeven's Hospital, Mercer's Hospital and St Patrick's Hospital (1747), on the other hand, actually began their working lives in purpose-built buildings, designed by architects, on the edges of the city (Figure 8).

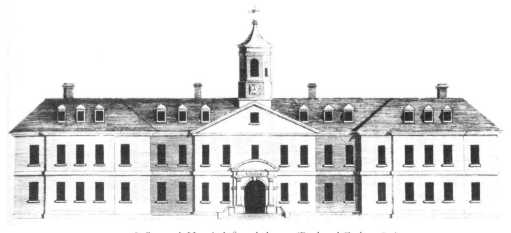

8 Steeven's Hospital, founded 1733. (Pool and Cash, 1780.)

Significantly, these latter examples were all founded by a committee formed to execute a legacy left by a single benefactor. Such an arrangement tended to allow the uncompromised execution of a single vision partly because enough capital was available to allow the acquisition of a large enough site and construction of a building more or less in one go. These two different trends of hospital foundation (appropriated domestic premises and purpose built), therefore, broadly followed the financial and social circumstances of their founders rather than any vastly differing methodology concerning treatment, admissions or administration. However, whereas Watson's *Almanack* informs us that the committees of Steeven's, Mercer's and St Patrick's were all dominated by members of society outside the medical and surgical professions, in the case of smaller hospitals, such as the Charitable Infirmary, the publication often failed to list any governors at all, publishing instead only the latter institutions' practitioners – surgeons, physicians and occasionally apothecaries. While it is perhaps unwise to read too much into this, the apparent absence of a group of governors suggests that a closer relationship between policy, organization and day-to-day treatment may have been more possible in the smaller hospitals.

Entry to a hospital's board of governors in the eighteenth century tended to require no specialized knowledge, but rather was dependent on privilege, social connection or simply the ability to make a donation in hard cash (Stevenson, 2000, p. 106). In Ireland, the Penal Laws had ensured that the upper echelons of society were dominated by Protestants and this was often reflected in the composition of hospital committees. There is, then, another possible difference between smaller and larger hospitals – the former may have been run by Roman Catholics. Unlike other professions in eighteenth-century Ireland, Catholics, while excluded from being educated in medicine and surgery, were not excluded from practising them. Indeed, it seems that the Charitable Infirmary had at least two among its founding surgeons (Logan and Martin, 1984). They, along with other Catholics, were presumably educated abroad, probably at one of the medical schools in Leyden in the Netherlands, Edinburgh or Paris. Significantly, the process whereby many small-scale domestic hospitals were transformed into larger, purpose built edifices often entailed the simultaneous acquisition of a similar type of aristocratic committee as existed at Steeven's, Mercer's or St Patrick's. This was most notable in the case of the Lying-in Hospital, but also occurred in the Meath Hospital (Gatenby, 1996) and the Lock Hospital (see below, Chapter 4).

Hospital practice in the eighteenth century

As stated above, surgeons were often at the forefront of establishing hospitals in the eighteenth century, a situation which would ultimately place surgery over medicine as the more progressive of the two practices in the eighteenth century. This was partly because, until the end of the nineteenth century, hospital patients were almost exclusively poor. Thus, the tactful conversations and negotiations concerning diagnosis and treatment which were characteristic of the physician's or surgeon's relationship with his fee-paying or upper-class clientele, were notably absent. In the hospital, patients were not clients but rather recipients of charity and therefore practitioners tended to have more control over them (Forty in King, ed., 1980, p. 74). The experience, almost always unpaid, gained in treating a concentrated and (for the most part) passive group of individuals in a hospital environment was beneficial not only to a practitioner's standing and reputation among fee-paying clients but also to his expertise. The practice of bodily examination, for example, which was unheard of in practitioner's dealings with upper-class, fee-paying clientele, inevitably helped the development of empirical, clinical medicine by loosening the restraints on the medical gaze. Such practices, however, were not without their critics and hospitals often attracted controversy. The eighteenth-century author Mary Wollstonecraft, for example, criticized patients' subordinate position in hospitals, suggesting that, 'everything appeared to be conducted for the accommodation of the medical men and their pupils who came to make experiments on the poor, for the benefit of the rich' (Wollestonecraft, 1798, in Kelly, ed., 1976, p. 117).

The creation of records and representations focused the new visibility permitted by hospital practice and made classification and comparisons possible. Hospital records containing very basic information, such as name, address (parish) and religion could allow prototypical statistical explorations into the geography of the city's poor. Meanwhile, similar techniques of observation, classification and representation, when applied to patients' bodies through the practice of dissection, allowed the creation of anatomical maps. Again, surgeons were at the forefront of these developments. It was they who taught anatomy in special schools through dissection, while physicians were still limited to examining external phenomena like the face, tongue and excrement (Stafford, 1993, p. 49). Dissection, however, was also a controversial pursuit, one which perhaps provided a focus in the popular imagination for some of the moral ambiguities connected to the bodily examination and indeed, the hospital. Peering intrusions, which provoked some anxiety when carried out on the living, passed into the realm of sacrilege when extended to the dead. Like other medical centres, such as Edinburgh and London, Dublin was the scene of periodic civil unrest concerning the practice and there are various accounts of rioting following body-snatching activities or the use of the bodies of executed criminals.

Male-midwifery and the founding of the Dublin Lying-in Hospital

Within the eighteenth-century medical and surgical hierarchy, obstetricians (also called 'men-midwives' or 'accoucheurs') occupied a lowly position. Theoretically a branch of surgery and therefore licensed to wield surgical instruments, throughout the eighteenth century male practitioners struggled to transform midwifery, a traditional craft dominated by women and riddled with superstition, into a notionally scientific profession administered by men (Donnison, 1977). This shift had social as well as gender implications. Female midwives were usually from modest backgrounds, whereas men-midwives like Mosse often had origins in the middle classes. It has been suggested that the combination of these circumstances meant that the nascent profession had palpable insecurities about the limits to its role and its status within society and resulted in a series of justifications produced to defend their profession and distance themselves from women practitioners. These included the writing of texts which condemned female midwives and deliberately exaggerated the dangers of childbirth. According to one eighteenth-century female midwife, this often went as far as concealing errors with 'a cloud of hard words and scientific jargon', while another suggested a façade of 'finished assurance' was adopted, to convince clients of great learning and expertise (Nihell, 1760 and Stone, 1737, both quoted in Donnison, 1977, p. 31).

The gender balance in midwifery gradually shifted over the course of the eighteenth century. Men-midwives, resplendent with coded knowledge and professional gravitas and armed with a variety of complicated looking surgical instruments, became a fashionable prerequisite, firstly, for upper-class birthings, then slowly throughout most of the other social classes, weakening the female midwife's position in each. Only the poor had tended to be insulated from this development partly because poor women were considered much more able to withstand the rigours of childbirth than their upper-class counterparts (Wolveridge, 1671). In fact, pregnancy was one of a series of conditions or types of patient, including children, lunatics, fever and venereal patients, which were initially barred from treatment at general hospitals such as the Charitable Infirmary, Steeven's Hospital or Mercer's Hospital. These exclusions presumably form the basis for the development of subsequent specialised hospitals like St Patrick's Hospital (1748, for lunatics), the Lock Hospital (for venereal patients) and the Cork Street Fever Hospital (1804). Institutionalized responses to childbirth, however, did exist elsewhere in Europe, most notably at the Hôtel Dieu, an institution which Mosse is thought to have visited in the 1740s, as part of the tour he took to 'improve' himself professionally (Wilde, 1846, p. 568).

As with the surgeons, hospital practice had certain benefits for the male-midwife. Firstly, the transferral of births to hospitals began to consolidate the subordinate position of the female midwife (Donnison, 1977, p. 27). Equally, as has been suggested above, the hospital could improve the practitioner's status and, especially in the case of the obstetrician, transform the ephemeral 'finished assurance' of expert knowledge into a more tangible manifestation: physical space in the city. In Dublin, however, a maternity hospital also seemed to have wider social implications. In a report entitled, *State of the Hospital*, published in November 1750, Benjamin Higgins (Mosse's colleague and first biographer) suggested some of Mosse's original reasons for founding the George's Lane hospital.

> [The women's] lodgings were generally in cold garrets open to every wind, or in damp cellars, subject to floods from excessive rains; destitute of attendance, medicines, and often of proper food, by which hundreds perished with their little infants … These distresses excited his compassion, and [Mosse] resolved no longer to delay his endeavours to establish an hospital for poor lying-in women … [H]e took a large house in George's-lane, which he furnished with beds and other necessaries, and opened the same on 15th of March, 1745.
> (Higgins quoted in Wilde, 1846, p. 568)

Earlier accounts, such as the following from 1745, emphasized the scheme's social and civic usefulness.

> As this hospital is solely designed for the use of such poor and distressed women as are not in circumstances to provide themselves at such time with a convenient place to lye-in, or with the common necessaries for persons in such a condition, by which means many poor

though honest and industrious women perish, and leave their helpless orphans a burthen to the public (notwithstanding they may at any hour have the best assistance in the physical way that this city affords), therefore, the directors of this hospital request that the public recommend none but such as truly merit the benefit of this most useful charity'.

(*Faulkner's Journal*, 23–26 March 1745)

The 'public burthen' of orphans had partly manifested itself in the necessity for the Foundling Hospital. Established in 1727 as part of the Poor House (1703) it had aimed to prevent 'exposure, death and actual murder of illegitimate children' and to bring up children in the Protestant faith, [and] thereby to strengthen and promote the Protestant interest in Ireland'. Despite these aspirations, this institution had almost immediately gained some of the negative associations of an *ancien régime* hospital: a vast and expensive container of squalid conditions, which ultimately degenerated into a site of 'unspeakable horrors' (Craig, 1992, p. 75) and where, of the 10,781 foundlings admitted between 1750 and 1760, *c.*3,800 (about 49 per cent) died. The reference to infanticide in the Foundling Hospital's mandate, however, was also taken up by Mosse as a justification for his Lying-in hospital which, 'would be a means not only of preserving the Lives, and relieving the Miseries of numberless Lying-in Women, but also preventing that most (unnatural) though too frequent Practice of abandoning or perhaps murdering new born Infants' (Royal Charter, 1756).

Better conditions and attending expertise would, it was hoped, decrease the numbers of mothers dying in childbirth. What is less clear, is precisely how the hospital could prevent the abandoning of children or their murder. However, the production of records – of who had given birth, to how many and when – would tend to make the abandoning or murdering of children more visible and identifiable. In June 1746, the *Dublin Journal* published a statistical account of the first year of the hospital, not only stressing its productivity through the numbers of successfully discharged patients, but also the regularity and exactitude of its records (see appendix 1: extracts from *Dublin Journal*).

> In this Hospital an exact Register is kept of all the Women when admitted and when discharged, from what places they come, and whose wives they are, and the Certificates of ministers, Church-wardens, and others recommending them for good Character and poverty; and of the

Children born whether Boys or Girls; and a faithful account is kept of the Money received and expended for the use of the Hospital.

(Dublin Journal, June 1746)

The precision of the records was subsequently acknowledged by no lesser person than Sir William Wilde, author of Ireland's first modern census and widely regarded as the father of modern statistics in Ireland. He commented that the hospital registry, from the period 1745 to 1755, which classified the patients' according to '[their] Ages, the parishes in Dublin and other parts of the kingdom from which they came, the class of society to which they belonged, the number of deliveries, results, and sex of births, and the mortalities of mothers and children, together with the number of twins' – represented one of the 'most interesting and earliest statistical tables on record' (Wilde, 1846, p. 577). He also suggested, moreover, that the Lying-in Hospital registry was 'better kept' than those of other hospitals from his own time, a hundred years later.

The form of the first Lying-in Hospital

In 1897, as part of a series of articles on the history of Dublin hospitals, the *Irish Builder* described the building (which was still extant) in George's Lane (later renamed South Great George's Street) where Mosse had originally established his hospital. It was a large three storey house with twelve rooms with a rear building containing two additional small wards with 'out-offices'. The whole ensemble stood 'back from the street', was approached by a narrow alley, and originally had a courtyard in front of it which had been long since filled up with other buildings (*Irish Builder,* March 1897, p. 59).

A similar account from 1846 suggested that the hospital's position 'opposite Fade-street', was still discernible on 'some of the old maps of the city' (Wilde, 1846, p. 569). Both accounts stress that the hospital was back from the street, implying that the building did not enjoy a public frontage. From these descriptions a number of possible sites around the vicinity can be discerned on Rocque's *Exact Survey*. None, however, can be conclusively identified (Figure 10). The most obvious site located directly opposite Fade Street, would seem to be refuted by the presence of the two small buildings to the rear, neither of which appear to correspond with Wilde's description of a 'three storey house' or the nineteenth-century illustration shown above (Figure 9). This confusion and indeed, the invisibility hinted by Wilde and the *Irish Builder,* is reinforced by Rocque's map. No site in the area is marked as a

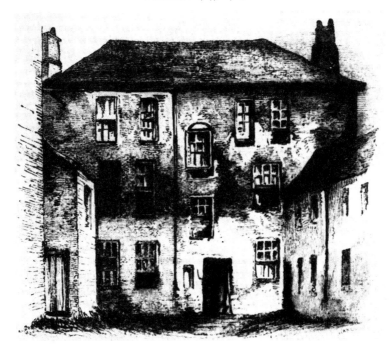

9 The original Lying-in Hospital building in the late-nineteenth century.

hospital, despite the fact that the Lying-in Hospital was operating there during the period when the *Exact Survey* was being prepared. In fact, Rocque chose to represent the not yet completed building at Great Britain Street as 'The Lying-in Hospital', a decision which perhaps explains its absence from George's Lane.

In the *Exact Survey*, Rocque employed a rudimentary classification system to describe the functions of the buildings he mapped. In this system back-land buildings, like those forming the Mosse's hospital, were identified as belonging to a class of 'Ware Houses, Stables &c.' effectively distinguishing them from 'Dwelling Houses', like the ones which fronted George's Lane itself. Evidence suggests that Mosse himself owned the 'Dwelling House' at the front of the Lying-in Hospital's site as well as the 'Backside Garden stable and coach House' ('Lease for the Property', 1745, RHR). According to Watson's *Almanack*, Mosse moved house from Dame Street to George's Lane sometime in 1746. Meanwhile, another contemporary publication differentiated between Mosse's 'house' and 'hospital' in its notice asking for the payment of arrears by benefactors, whom it instructed to pay 'Joseph Miller, at the Hospital … or to Doctor Mosses at his House in George's Lane' (*Faulkner's Journal*, 5–8 July 1746).

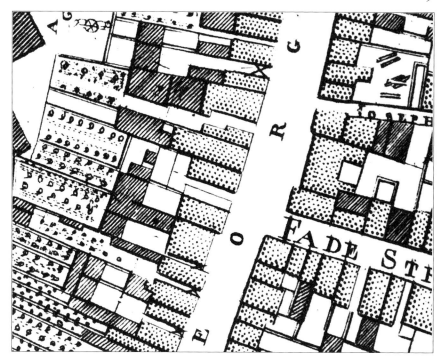

10 The locale of the original Lying-in Hospital at George's Lane.
(John Rocque, *Exact Survey*, 1756.)

The domestic arrangement of a house with a hospital at the rear of the same plot perhaps fitted the status and resources of a surgeon/obstetrician whose modest project had not yet achieved official sanction or widespread recognition. Yet it also displayed a hierarchy. Mosse's house formed part of the public realm. His hospital, on the other hand, was in the back-lands, in a series of spaces normally reserved for services and production, but inhabited all over the city by the poor. While spatial differentiation according to medical needs was still in its infancy, Mosse's arrangement was differentiated socially. In fact, the relative invisibility of Mosse's first hospital contrasted with the Charitable Infirmary, Mercer's, Steeven's, St Patrick's and even the Lock Hospital (at Rainsford Street), all of which enjoyed at least some visual presence from the street and, moreover, are all clearly marked on Rocque's *Exact Survey*.

The controversies of a maternity hospital

If there was a popular uneasiness associated with hospitals in general, as sites of ritualistic practice and places 'to make experiments on the poor', then this

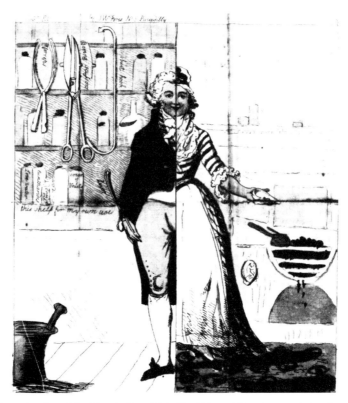

11 An illustration from John Blunt's *Man-Midwifery Dissected* (London, 1793) showing a variety of surgical instruments. Mosse himself possessed a wide range of surgical and obstetrical implements; these included: two dissecting knives, two pairs of scissors, two tapping instruments, five silver instruments, a large midwifery instrument, two hooks with ivory handles, seven small instruments, a pair of 'head pincers' and, perhaps most intriguingly, 'an artificial lying-in woman'. The 'head pincers' were bought by William Collum, the future Master of the Lying-in Hospital, for three shillings. The 'artificial lying-in woman' was bought for £2 10s. by a Mr O'Donnell whose connection to obstetrics remains unknown. ('Auctioneer's book regarding Dr Mosse's auction' in Rotunda Hospital Records.)

was perhaps intensified in the case of a maternity hospital. Some contemporary texts accused the practice of man-midwifery of being at best quackery and at worst fundamentally immoral. One such harangue, written by a John Blunt in the late-eighteenth century, sought to expose what the author considered to be the immoral tendency of those men who practised midwifery. Evocatively titled, *Man-Midwifery Dissected; or the Obstetric Family Instructor ... containing a Display of the Management of Every Class of Labours by Men and Boy Midwives; also of their cunning, indecent and cruel Practices ... proving that Man-midwifery is a personal, a domestic, and a national Evil*, the cover of the publication was illustrated with a hermaphroditic figure bisected into a male and female half (Figure 11). Behind the female half is a stove, within which we can just see a tiny figure indicating either a botched delivery or abortion while behind the male half, a series of shelves hold bottles marked 'Cream of Violets' and 'Love Water' as well as a ferocious set of surgical instruments.

An obstetrician's notebook (contained in the Rotunda Hospital Records), entitled 'Miscellanea Medica', signed 'D.M.M., 1750' and possibly written by Mosse himself, provides a graphic insight into the experiences of a male-midwife operating in the mid-eighteenth century. Its meticulously indexed notes and observations are symptomatic of the growing concern amongst practitioners for empirical and scientific techniques. Each case is numbered, the woman's name given (or listed simply as 'Poor Lying-in Woman') and is followed by remarks on the delivery. Most cases are entered as normal, 'Natural Delivery'. Some, however, note complications which, as the following excerpts testify, were not always relieved by the obstetrician's expertise or, indeed, his use of instruments.

> Case No. 23 – Poor Woman in the Barracks, 30 July 1754.
>
> First Child – the head engaged in the pelvis – had been 36 hours in labour – tried my new invented affair which did not answer much after it – brought the head by the forceps – the uterus inflamed was relieved by bleeding, repeated clysters and fomenting the belly with emollients.
>
> Case No. 147 Nurse Bryan's daughter
>
> The uterus still gave way before my hand and retreated quite up into the belly as it were, I could not imagine how this should happen – till after I had brought away everything, on putting up my hand I found the uterus fairly torn from the vagina at the back part – This amazed me still the more as I had wrought with the utmost caution and as I thought, and used very little force [next part crossed out] but the putrid child had certainly caused a suppuration. She died in half an hour. I was immensely shocked that I should have interfered, and not rather have left her to the pains, which I certainly should have done, for there was at the time I saw her no urgent necessity for delivering her. But I thought her delivery was the luckiest thing that could have happened to her and so it certainly would have proved if the she had either been left to nature, or it could have been done without injury.

> Every labour and abortion, should be trusted to the natural pains, unless something very urgent requires the assistance of my hand.
>
> ('Miscellanea Medica', 1750, pp 220–2)

These kind of messy scenes perhaps also generated the need to locate the hospital away from the public realm and conceal it behind the façade of a respectable middle-class residence. Elsewhere, throughout the eighteenth century, critics of obstetrics often concentrated on the sexual improprieties alleged to be connected with the practice. Francis Foster's *Thoughts for the Times but Chiefly on the Profligacy of Our Women*, published in London in 1779, suggested midwifery gave 'the enemy access to the very citadel of female virtue', a breach of intimacy which was made all the more perilous when combined with the 'unnatural lusts' that pregnant women of all classes were thought to succumb to (Stafford, 1993, p. 307). Meanwhile, Elizabeth Nihell in her *Treatise on the Art of Midwifery* extended Foster's criticism to hospitals, where she observed women were in danger of being 'harassed' by male students (quoted in Campbell-Ross, 1986, p. 160).

In fact, this last criticism found an echo in Dublin later in the century when Mosse's original vision of the hospital as having a teaching role – 'in order to prevent gentlemen going abroad for instruction' (quoted in Wilde, 1846) – was challenged by William Collum (Master of the hospital from 1766 to 1773), who suggested such an arrangement could result in a breach of modesty for all concerned. He argued that, '[i]f woman's frailty was well-known to the eighteenth century, then young men were not to be needlessly tempted to lustful thoughts' (Collum, Dublin, 1770). In 1771, Frederick Jebb, who would ultimately replace Collum as Master of the hospital, published a response. While strenuously arguing for the necessity of teaching in the hospital, Jebb, however, also alluded to the fact that Mosse himself had been the target of some criticism and allegations but perhaps significantly, failed to state on what charges.

> But alas! not even the Prudence and Wisdom, or the Virtue of Dr Mosse were sufficient to defend him from the Tax that is levied on Merit. Pelted both in public and in private with Obloquy and Scandal, treated with every Species of insolent Dissidence.
>
> (Jebb, Dublin, 1771, pp 21–2)

Whatever the dubious connotations associated with a maternity hospital, Mosse's original site at George's Lane had perhaps compounded the problem.

While the back-land building had nothing explicit within its external form to merit the description, it had formerly contained a theatre, called The New Booth, one of a number of similar small, informal theatrical venues which had sprung up throughout the seventeenth and early eighteenth centuries around the area. After opening in 1730, The New Booth was closed down just before 1745 amidst allegations of scandal and turpitude concerning the 'exhibitionist tendencies' of its owner and leading lady Madame Violante, 'the Italian rope-walker' (Boydell, 1988, p. 292). In a climate of popular suspicion and lack of understanding of the medical, surgical and obstetrical professions, its reopening as a maternity hospital may have been considered not so much as a break from its former activities but rather a continuation: in the hidden back-lands of the city, female anatomy was still being exposed to a limited audience.

Mosse's first use of theatre

At the same time, however, as the medical gaze and its correlative the anatomical theatre was being viewed with a mixture of anxiety and mistrust, Mosse was appealing to the other type of theatre as a source not only of revenue but also of legitimacy. Drawing upon a precedent where the proceedings of the first performance in 1742 of Handel's *Messiah* were distributed between the Charitable Infirmary and the Mercer's Hospital, Mosse decided to stage a theatrical production. Within six weeks of the hospital's opening, a morality play by Ambrose Philip called *The Distressed Mother* was staged in the Smock Alley Theatre. Perhaps significantly, the same phrase 'distressed mother' also appeared in early notices in publications such as *Faulkner's Journal* (and indeed, Mosse's application for a royal charter in 1752) when describing the hospital's activities. Its use in the two different contexts of reportage and stage-craft, effectively blurred the boundaries between fact and fiction. If the hospital skulked around the ill-lit precincts of the city, a periodic target of allegations, then the idealised world of theatre could be used to produce another, public façade.

The approach worked. *The Distressed Mother* made £150 in ticket receipts, prompted a number of citizens to subscribe £15 per annum and ultimately allowed ten new beds to be created at the hospital. It was followed by another play entitled *Cato*, before Mosse turned to music when Handel's *Esther* was given a gala performance in aid of the hospital at the Fishamble Street Music Hall in February 1746. In the meantime, while the exact content of the first play remains unknown, idealized representations of motherhood were to become a recurring theme in the subsequent history of the hospital. Moreover, just as in the eighteenth-century theatre, where the division between actors and audience was not always distinct or given a clear spatial threshold – until 1747, for example, spectators could still stand on stage during performances (Mooney and White in Dickson, ed., 1987, p. 6) – the relationship between Mosse's hospital building and the public realm may have been more complex and ambiguous than it at first appears.

The prize draws for fund-raising lotteries, for instance, often took place at the hospital in George's Lane causing, 'no little excitement amongst the inmates' (Kirkpatrick and Jellet, 1914, p. 16). This suggests that certain moments of contact existed between the patients and a ticket-buying public, a relationship which would develop in the new hospital. A poem, written by the Revd William Dunkin, to be spoken immediately before *The Distressed Mother* was performed, detailed the uses of the hospital and those who were to inhabit it. It invoked amongst other things, images of moral rectitude and the beauties of motherhood; 'the tender Mother and the faithful Wife', 'blissful Beauties and unspotted Truth,' and 'Ye chaste Maids, who ripening, hope to prove, the Sweets of Wedlock, and the Fruits of Love' (*Dublin Journal*, 1745). The contrast between this and the case-notes of D.M.M. could not be more acute.

The colonial landscape

In 1748, Emily, countess of Kildare, gave birth to George, the first of her nineteen children. Others followed in rapid succession; William, 1749, Caroline, 1750, Emily, 1752 and so on until the last, another George (the first having died in 1765) in 1773. When she suspected her confinement was close, Emily usually moved to Leinster House in Dublin to prepare for the birth and, following aristocratic fashion, always had a male midwife in attendance (Tillyard, 1995, p. 231). Mosse was one of only three obstetricians licensed by the Royal College of Physicians in Dublin at that time. Accordingly, it is perhaps no surprise to learn that when, four years later, Mosse made his successful application for a Royal Charter for his hospital, 'the Right Honourable, James, earl of Kildare' was listed as a vice-president, taking his place alongside the lord lieutenant, the duke of Dorset (president); Father in God, George Stone, archbishop of Armagh and an esteemed collection of other Irish noble families as the hospital's governors and guardians. Indeed, while many of the other governors were elected 'for the time being', the earls of Kildare were honoured with governorship 'for ever' (*Royal Charter*, 1752). Mosse's association with Kildare (elevated to duke of Leinster in November 1766) lasted the rest of his life.

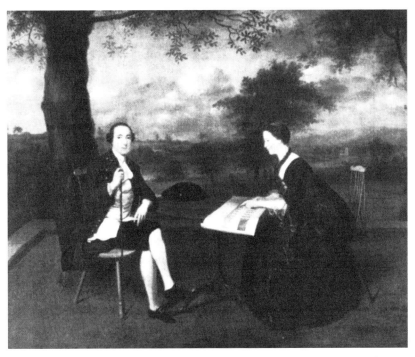

12 James and Emily, earl and countess of Kildare, depicted in an imaginary landscape based on their estate at Carton, County Kildare. (Arthur Devis, 1755.)

While the Kildares were an old and established Irish aristocratic family and Mosse was the product of later colonial settlement, both had benefited from the accession of William of Orange. As the turbulences of the seventeenth century quelled after the defeat of James II's forces at the battle of the Boyne, a period of relative calm and prosperity descended on Ireland. Mosse's father, having served as royal chaplain to William, was rewarded by being made rector of Maryborough (Portlaoise today), a town which lay at the heart of the first Protestant plantation of Ireland, the Leix-Offaly plantation of 1556. Bartholomew Mosse was born there around 1712 and grew up in the town. Meanwhile, the settlements following the peace in 1690 consolidated the superior position of Protestant landowners – whether newly arrived planter or from an older family like Kildare – by transferring vast tracts of the Irish countryside into their hands. This last development, however, was partly made possible by the colonizers' attitude towards the qualities and characteristics of land and space. The *Down Survey*, executed by Sir William Petty, surveyor general of Ireland, in 1652, exemplified what has been called, 'foreign land-measuring, classifying and appropriation techniques' (O'Kane, 2000, p. 8).

Inevitably this, the first scientific cartography of Ireland, presupposed negation. Not only did the survey facilitate the speedy transfer of land to Cromwell's soldiers, adventurers and supporters, the imposition of an abstract, rational system of measurement and representation began to dissolve indigenous Irish social and cultural connections to land and replace them with English ideas of ownership and property rights. The appearance of the big house in the landscape confirmed the colonial presence. Originally constructed primarily with a military function, to withstand attack and facilitate the relay of communications, the new-found peace and subjugation of the enemy allowed the colonizer's architecture to transform itself accordingly from mute defensive enclaves into more active manipulators of the land. The tower house was gradually replaced by the country villa, with each successive architectural transformation shedding more of its overt military origins while retaining a symbolic and increasingly economic dominance over its hinterland.

In the *terra firma*, the land on the Italian peninsula conquered by the Venetian Republic in the sixteenth century, the villas designed by the architect Andrea Palladio and his colleagues had occupied a similar position. There, as in Ireland, the colonizers had assumed an existing landscape of chaos and disorder and a divine right, perhaps even obligation, to transform it. A symbiotic relationship between villa and associated estate provided the means to harness the potential of inanimate land and space to create a productive entity. The architecture of the villa, its size, form and decoration, embodied the wealth derived from the science of agriculture (Cosgrove, 1993, p. 250).

Introduced into Britain by the British architect Inigo Jones in the seventeenth century, Palladian architecture was subject to a series of political appropriations. Initially used by James VI (of Scotland) & I (of Great Britain) to bolster his visions of the divine right of kings, ironically, by the eighteenth century, Palladianism had become the favoured motif of the Whigs, a party dominated by the anti-royalist ideologies of John Locke. The Whigs have been described as 'Parliamentarians, some even Republicans, who were positive Protestants and in the extreme, Puritans' (Tavernor, 1991, p. 151). Their ascendancy into power at the end of the seventeenth century, had, by the early eighteenth, crystallized into an oligarchy. Whiggish appropriation of Palladian architecture, however, went beyond the vagaries of mere stylistic preference. Rather its associations of productivity resonated with a contemporary ideology of improvement. Here, through the medium of transformed and regulated land, an estate passed from being regarded merely as an inheritance, to being calculated as an opportunity for investment and ultimately as a source of greatly increased profits. Traditional 'social relations which stood in the way of this kind of modernisation were then steadily and ruthlessly broken down' (Williams, 1985, pp 60–1). One of the 'social relations' alluded to here, concerned the common ownership of land. Parliamentary enclosure, from the second quarter of the eighteenth century to the first quarter of the nineteenth, facilitated the appending of this common land to the estates of the big houses. The scale of these interventions was huge: almost six million acres (2.4m ha) of land were appropriated – about a quarter of all cultivated land – through nearly four thousand Acts, mainly by the politically dominant landowners (Williams, 1985, p. 96).

While originally applying to the commons of the Great British mainland, enclosure bore a close similarity to colonial intervention: a dissolving or negation of previous property relations. By the 1720s, a period of prosperity for the propertied classes, inspired partly by the Whig administration in Britain, was echoed in Ireland. Like its counterpart across the water, this manifested itself in a country-house building boom. Castletown House in County Kildare is considered one of the most magnificent of this period (Craig, 1992, p. 101; Foster, 1988, p. 191). Designed by Alessandro Galilei in 1722 for William Conolly, the speaker of the Irish House of Commons, it is a vast Palladian villa displaying the typical arrangement of a centre piece flanked by two pavilions. A few years later, at Carton, an adjacent estate, the Protestant immigrant architect Richard Cassels, produced a similar, if more prosaic, arrangement for the earl of Kildare. Irish adoption of the architecture of the Palladian villa, tended to be purer and more complete than in England. Here, the farm-buildings tended to be integrated into the overall architectural composition, an arrangement which not only more clearly emphasized utility and productivity, but also reiterated the coloniser's role in 'creating' the land (Foster, 1988, p. 193).

The Protestant Anglo-Irish tended to be 'Whig almost by definition' (O'Kane, 2000, p. 12). Historical experience had made them so. The class owed its privileged position to the successes of Cromwell and William of Orange and, despite the peace, the continued Protestant domination of Ireland was not entirely certain. The restless spectre of returning Catholic Jacobites still lingered on the fringes of possibility. This, when combined with an indigenous Catholic majority on the island, effectively precluded any Anglo-Irish complacency. Accordingly, while in England the changes in the countryside met with some resistance from a rear-guard of conservative British landowners, in Ireland, there was little aristocratic opposition: Whiggish ideals of improvement blended easily with the colonial project. By the 1730s, the practicalities of transforming and remaking the land were being avidly discussed in the Dublin Society, a voluntary association designed to promote economic activities and the major medium for transmitting new farming ideas (Dickson, 2000, pp 124–5). However, as well as debating, discussing and disseminating new theories and techniques designed to make fertile, propagate and cultivate land and crops, the Society's members also investigated wider societal concerns such as unemployment amongst the lower classes and, significantly, the ever critical question of population on the island. Amongst its members, it counted Bartholomew Mosse.

Popular resistance to agrarian reform did exist in Ireland, however, manifesting itself in shadowy militant groups such as the Whiteboys and the Oakboys, whose insurrectionary activities periodically troubled landlords throughout the second half of the century. Indeed, as is hinted above, the fecundity of the improved landscape was simultaneously dependent on dispossession and exclusion. As landholding became more subject to market forces, thousands of smaller tenant farmers and peasants were transformed into wage labourers, while simultaneously, advances in farming technology meant that often their labour was no longer needed. Released from the land, many of them drifted towards urban centres contributing massively to Dublin's population growth throughout the second half of the century. Meanwhile, enclosure and the polarisation of wealth resulted in abrupt disjunctions between the fertility and abundance of improved land, which contained at its heart the exotic trees, groves and shrubbery of the demesne's pleasure gardens, and the barren, treeless 'monochrome environment' of the unimproved landscape (O'Kane, 2000, p. 2). On the British mainland, the radical nature of these transformations tended to be obscured by a patina of timelessness and permanence; 'ancient or ancient-seeming titles and houses [which] offered the illusion of a society still determined by obligation and traditional relations between social orders' (Williams, 1985, p. 60). Palladian architecture, disseminated through contemporary pattern books like Colen Campbell's *Vitruvius Britannica*, cloaked radical changes with the 'antique simplicity' of classical virtue (Tavernor, 1991, p. 153).

As the transformation of peasants into wage labourers in Ireland took place in a colonial context, 'on a landscape only recently won and insecurely held' the Anglo-Irish landowners' search for legitimacy perhaps assumed an additional urgency. It has been suggested, for example, that Anglo-Irish anxieties manifested themselves in an elaborate building programme which was psychologically necessary but often extravagant far beyond their economic wherewithal. As well as building to convince themselves they had been there a long time, they also built to convince themselves they would remain (Foster, 1988, p. 194). Initially at least, this programme was isolationist and introspective; 'within the walls of the demesne, the Anglo-Irish ascendancy constructed their visions of an Irish Utopia' (O'Kane, 2000, p. 2). Here, according to many of the painted representations of the time, they could wander through landscapes devoted to the pursuit of pleasure and indulge in a variety of liberal entertainments. Often they were accompanied in this endeavour, not only by carefully composed images of cheerfully toiling, acquiescent peasants, but also, in the distance, by the stately gaze of the country villa, symbolic centre of this ordered and productive world.

Kildare House: rural harmony in the city

When Robert Fitzgerald, nineteenth earl of Kildare, died in February 1744, he was succeeded by his son, James. One of the new earl's first acts was to buy a plot for a town house in Dublin, to replace the existing residence in Suffolk Street. He chose a site on the eastern fringes of the city. Two well-known stories are often cited in connection with the building. One; when questioned by a friend over the remoteness of his choice of site, Kildare replied, with reference to his importance within Irish society, that '[t]hey will follow me wherever I go' (Craig, 1992, p. 133). The other; also concerning the site, explains its location as a compromise between Kildare, who wanted a town house and his architect, Richard Cassels, who wanted a country one. Brought to Ireland in 1727 under the patronage of Sir Gustavus Hume, Cassels' arrival dovetailed neatly with the building boom. He acquired a reputation as one of the country's most eminent architects after producing a string of houses in the Palladian style: Hazelwood House in County Sligo, Powerscourt House in County Wicklow, Carton House in County Kildare, Bessborough House in County Kilkenny as well as Tyrone House, Kildare House, Lord Bective's House in Smithfield and a variety of smaller houses throughout the city of Dublin. He also produced a few public buildings in Dublin mainly in Trinity College: the Printing House (1734), the Dining Hall (1745–9) and the tower and dome which he added to the old Chapel (Craig, 1992, p. 131).

Kildare's move and Cassels' series of commissions for town houses reflected a new aristocratic interest in building in the city. This began with an escape from the overcrowded old town and the creation of its antidote: a series of wide and generously proportioned suburbs such as the Jervis Estate which was located across the river on the city's north side. These were built speculatively with streets and squares laid out, mostly on land formerly belonging to abbeys and monasteries, before being divided into individual plots and bought and sold. It has been suggested that some of these new streets resembled the spaciousness of rural estates, with a similar desire for light and space ultimately becoming embodied within the Georgian terraced house itself (Campbell, 1998, p. 17). A similar phenomenon has been observed in eighteenth-century London where the interiors of architects such as Robert Adam created the illusion of spaciousness with top-lit staircases securing a light and airy feel and reception rooms designed *en suite* to provide long vistas (Porter, 1996, pp 114–15).

A specific London example effectively deepens this argument. It has been suggested that 20, St James's Square embodies a conscious attempt to transpose an idealised vision of the countryside into the realm of an eighteenth-century London terraced house. Here, the space, fabric, decoration and iconography of the building were used to reaffirm the 'Virgilian myth of man's harmony with nature' (Olley, 1990, p. 53). Most striking are the two paintings by Richard Wilson, which probably hung in one of the drawing rooms and which depicted bucolic scenes from the owner, Sir Watkin Williams Wynn's rural estate. Within them, we are treated to a familiar blend of a picturesque landscape punctuated by happy peasants, gentry at leisure and supervised, as ever, by the distant mansion. The presence of such harmonious scenes in the drawing room of an urban terrace, perhaps indicates an aspiration that the natural order and hierarchy of the demesne would ultimately find itself transplanted into the city.

For the most illustrious in Dublin, the search for a citified rural life took them, rather like the French *hôtels* of the late seventeenth century (after the return of the court from Versailles to Paris), to the periphery of the city. The location of Tyrone House (begun in 1740) and Kildare House (begun in 1745) on the eastern edges of urban Dublin, for example, allowed the construction of a type of architecture similar to the villa and therefore a closer approximation of the comforts of the demesne (Figure 2). Like their rural counterparts, the large scale and luxurious decoration of these buildings absorbed and displayed the profits created by the shifts in the rural economy.

It has been suggested that the plan of Kildare House was reminiscent to that of an Irish country residence, where equal attention was paid to both of its long elevations; '[t]here is no "back": the eastern front though plainer, is as

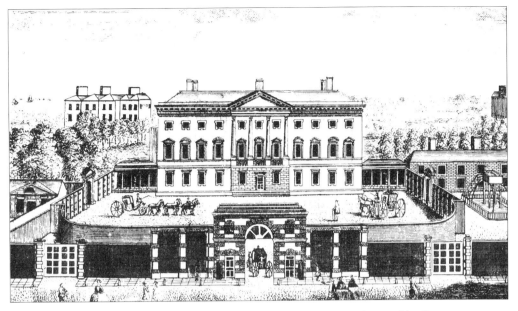

13 Kildare House west front. (Vignette from John Rocque, *A Survey of the City, Harbour, Bay and Environs of Dublin*, 1757.)

formal as the western and to many tastes superior' (Craig, 1992, p. 133). The building's layout, however, seems more reminiscent of the French *hôtel*, with an elaborate public front and hard courtyard, designed to be seen from the city, and a garden at the rear, in proximity to the countryside, and designed to be viewed from the house (Figure 13 and 14). The latter quality is perhaps suggested by the arrangement of the rear apartments. These are laid out in an *enfilade* system where one moves directly from room to room through a series of aligned doors located close to the windows. The purpose of the *enfilade* (a common arrangement in the French *hôtel*) was to allow a promenade which addressed the garden while enjoying the comforts of interior space.

On Rocque's *Exact Survey*, the cartographer marked the garden of Leinster House with a diverse variety of planting arrangements and, moreover, felt compelled to name the plot, 'Kildare House and Garden' (Figure 14). It was in this enclosed space, an urban surrogate of the rural demesne's pleasure garden, that the latter's activities would continue anew in the city as Kildare House acquired an enduring reputation as a house of hospitality and entertainment. There, one could witness, in the setting of an idealized landscape, an equally ideal and fantastic world of masques, plays and sundry *jeux*, designed to captivate and enthral both audience and participants – a

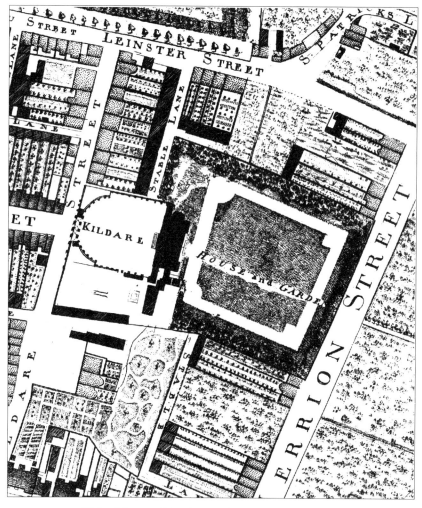

14 Kildare House and Gardens on the eastern fringes of the city
(John Rocque's *Exact Survey*, 1756).

setting which seemed to justify Henry Fielding's argument that a contemporary intensification of theatricality in everyday life had significantly altered the boundaries between fact and representation.

> The world hath often been compared to the theatre; and many grave writers, as well as poets, have considered human life as a great drama, resembling, in almost every particular, those scenical representations, which Thespis is first reported to have invented and which have been since received with so much approbation and delight in all polite

countries. This though hath been carried so far, and became so general, that some words proper to theatre, and which were, at first, metaphorically applied to the world, are now indiscriminately and literally spoken of both: thus stage and scene are by common use as familiar to us, when we speak of life in general, as when we confine ourselves to dramatic performances; and when we mention transactions behind the curtain, St James is more likely to occur in thoughts than Drury Lane.

(Fielding, 1794, p. 299)

Kildare House and the new Lying-in Hospital: a comparison

On 25 August 1748, seven months after Emily Fitzgerald gave birth to her first baby and just under three-and-a-half years after the opening of the Lying-in Hospital in George's Lane, Mosse signed a lease to himself, 'his heirs and assigns, for lives renewable for ever, at the yearly rent of £70', for a piece of ground of 'four acres and nineteen perches, from W. Naper Esq.'

> A plot or piece of ground situate on the north side of Great Brittain-street [*sic*], bounded on the north by ground belonging to Mr. Thomas Shanley; on the east by ground belonging to the Right Hon. Luke Gardiner Esq., now held by Mr. Nicholson; on the south side by Great Brittain street; and on the west, partly by the house, yard, backside, and garden belonging to and now held by Lord Mount Garret, and partly by ground belonging to the Right Hon. Luke Gardiner, Esq., now held by Mr. Butterly and Mr. Kenny.
>
> (*Irish Builder*, December 1893, p. 268)

Mosse's first act on taking possession, was to have the plot enclosed by a high wall. Within this enclosure, the 'New Pleasure Gardens' were laid-out with Robert Stevenson, the first gardener being paid £34 2*s*. 6*d*. between 1748 and 1750, 'for his trouble in designing on paper and staking out the New Gardens, directing and planting, ordering and dressing the different particulars' (RHR). Rocque's *Exact Survey* reveals close similarities between the site of the new Lying-in Hospital and that of Kildare House (Figure 2). The hospital, perched on the northern edge of the city, echoed Kildare House's position on the city's eastern fringes. The apparent relationship between house, garden, city and countryside was also strikingly similar: a hard courtyard edge addressed the city, while on the other side, a planned and ordered garden was bounded by a wall which screened the countryside. Yet the Lying-in Hospital's relationship with the city, unhindered by Kildare House's long, walled outer courtyard, was more immediate. It stood closer to the public realm, an arrangement which was perhaps intensified by its flanking wings which seemed to reach out on its southern side to embrace the streetscape. Like the rural villa's close attachment with its pleasure garden and more distant, but equally potent relationship with the rest of its estate, the Lying-in Hospital provided a visible presence in the city which embodied productivity and perhaps symbolized an active role in the creation of an urban

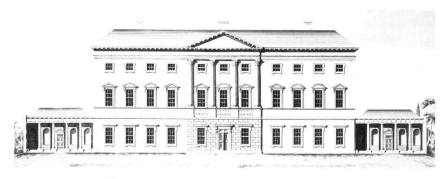

15 Kildare House west elevation. (Thomas Cunningham, 1790.)

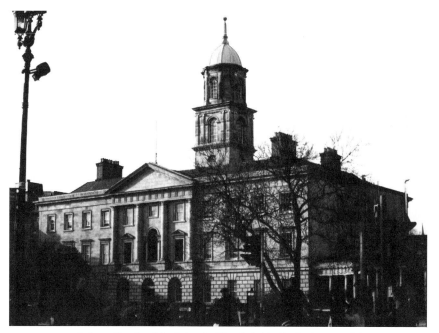

16 Front façade of the Lying-in Hospital. (Author's photograph.)

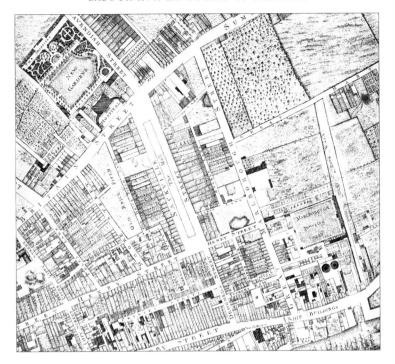

17 The hospital in its urban context, with Sackville Mall (middle) and Marlborough Gardens (lower right) in 1756. On the plan of the hospital note that the curved wings on the street-side of the building are not yet repeated on the garden side. Compare with Figure 26. (John Rocque, *Exact Survey*, 1756.)

equivalent of those harmonious landscapes of acquiescent peasants and benevolent aristocrats.

The parallels between the site layouts of Kildare House and the Lying-in Hospital were echoed in architectural form. Some observers have suggested that the Palladian form of the hospital looked more like the 'palace of a nobleman rather than a hospital', whereas Maurice Craig is more explicit in acknowledging the similarities, describing the hospital as 'not unlike [Kildare] House with a three storey tower and cupola perched on top' (1992, p. 143; Figures 15 and 16). As well as sharing Cassels as the architect, the two buildings also had tradesmen in common including Henry Darley 'mason and stonecutter'; John Semple, bricklayer; Alexander Brennan, plumber etc.

The lack of invoices from Cassels in the hospital records, moreover, may indicate that he provided his services free of charge. While a friendship between himself and Mosse, cemented by a series of late-night drinking sessions in a tavern in Fishamble Street, has been well-documented – 'they sacrificed much to Bacchus' (Gilbert, 1902–16, pp 314–16) – the architect was presumably financially supported by other clients and patrons, and most likely, the earl of Kildare. Cassels was working for Kildare at the same time as the hospital was being designed. His untimely death in the library at Carton in 1751, around the same time as the construction of the hospital commenced, led to the appointment of John Ensor as the architect in charge of completing the building. He was paid £262 9s. 6d. for his services.

There were, however, several differences between the architecture of Kildare House and the Lying-in Hospital. Most obvious was the hospital's three-storey tower and cupola, which Craig described as 'not very convincingly integrated with the substructure' (1992, p. 143). It did, however, place the hospital within a genre of institutional buildings in the city including the Royal Hospital, Kilmainham, Steeven's Hospital and Trinity College all of which were equipped with towers to announce their presence over the skyline. The Lying-in Hospital's place in this typology would have been even more emphatically expressed when originally surmounted by a gilded cradle, crown and ball, which was taken down later in the century due to fears of instability. In fact, Mosse also intended to embellish the tower with a chiming clock and a set of bells, but after complaints by 'neighbouring ladies' this was also curtailed. Perhaps more intriguing was an unexecuted scheme to construct a telescope and observatory in the tower perhaps conceived by Mosse as another potential money-making scheme. Less evident but perhaps more significant, the *enfilade* arrangement at the rear of Kildare House, was not replicated at the Lying-in Hospital, indicating a subtle difference in the relationship between building and garden: rather than viewing the garden from the house, the house was designed to be viewed from the garden. By 1764, this relationship had intensified with the arrival of two colonnaded wings, extending from the building to embrace the garden and mirroring those found on the city side and effectively equipping the hospital with two public fronts (compare Figure 17 with Figure 26).

Landscapes of pleasure

At about the same time Mosse was leasing his plot at Great Britain Street, another development was taking place in the vicinity. Between 1748 and 1750, to the east of the Jervis Estate, the property developer Luke Gardiner widened Drogheda Street 'on its west side until it was 150 feet (45.7m) from house to house', demolishing many houses 'not yet three quarters of a century old' and

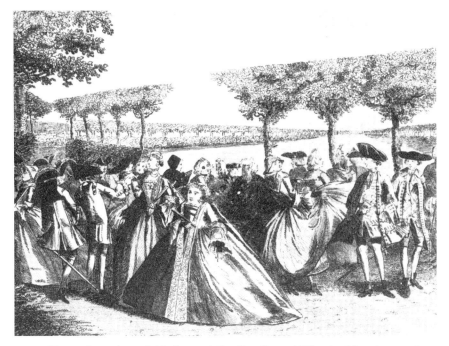

18 'Taste, à-la-mode 1745', Marlborough Bowling Green. (*Hibernian Magazine*, 1790.)

foregoing their rent revenues in the process (Walsh in Dickson, ed., 1987, p. 33). Gardiner renamed the street after the English statesman and aristocrat, Lionel Sackville, first duke of Dorset and twice lord lieutenant of Ireland. Soon, the building plots laid-out around it began to fill up with a series of upper-class residents. Sackville Street's conspicuous girth is illustrated in Rocque's *Exact Survey* (Figure 17). One thousand and fifty feet long (320m), it is at least twice as wide as any of the surrounding streets. Down its middle there was an enclosed pedestrian area called 'The Mall' which was ornamented on its perimeter by a series of lamps and obelisks and may have involved Cassels in its design and laying-out (Curran, 1947, p. 5). It soon became one of the city's favoured resorts of parade, where, 'the Dublin belles and *macaronies* of 1750; and the loungers of the north side of the city vied with those of the south, who strutted within the sunk fences and dirty ditches of St Stephen's-green' (Wilde, 1846, p. 580).

It has been suggested that the density of population and relative constraints of space in the city of London forced the development of substitute social spaces outside the home (Porter, 1994, pp 114–15). Streets, squares, shops, theatres, arcades and clubs became new public arenas and allowed new forms

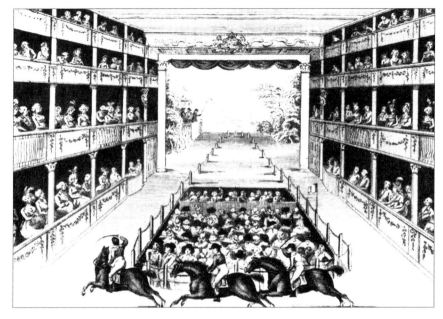

19 Interior of Theatre Royal. (*Hibernian Magazine*, November, 1795.)

of social life to develop. As the description of Sackville Mall and St Stephen's Green above hints, these new social relations were characterized by acts of display.

'Taste, à-la-mode', for example, a depiction of Marlborough Gardens in 1745, printed in the *Hibernian Magazine* in 1790, shows a typically flamboyant collection of hooped skirts, elaborate coat-tails and swords (Figure 18). Everyone in the print is either engaged in looking or being looked at. Similarly, the eighteenth-century theatre was often as much about the spectators' performance of gossiping, flirting and flaunting fashion, as it was about the performance on stage. A perspective of the interior of the Theatre Royal in Crow Street in 1795 depicts a pony race taking part on a course laid out around the pit and passing through the *proscenium arch* (the formal device which frames the opening between the stage and the auditorium; Figure 19). Upper class spectators inhabit rows of boxes at opposite sides of the theatre. From here they can not only view the race but also those persons sitting in the galleries across from them. The most remarkable aspect of this illustration, however, is its similarity to a perspective view of Sackville Street and Mall produced in 1752 (Figure 20). Here, strollers leisurely meander through and around the enclosed Mall (which echoes the form of the race course). In place of the theatre boxes, however, the houses of Sackville Street's blank windows gaze

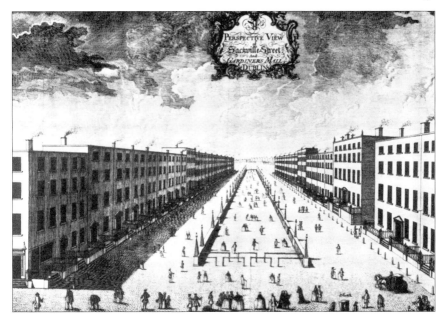

20 A perspective view of Sackville Street and Gardiner's Mall. (Oliver Grace, *c*.1752.)

down at the street's activities and across at each other. But like the theatre, this gaze is not mono-directional.

The figures who inhabit the street, gossiping or simply staring, can catch glimpses of the houses' interiors beyond the prosaic and uniform façades. More specifically, their eye is drawn to the ceilings of the *piano nobile*. The section of the house and its relationship with the street allows the stuccodore's art to express the owner's wealth and taste in a florid riot of plaster work while the remainder of the room remains invisible to the public realm. Those who inhabited the houses opposite, however, could perhaps witness considerably more.

To the list of new social spaces emerging from the urban condition, we can add the commercial pleasure garden. In 1764, John Bush described a visit to Mosse's New Pleasure Gardens, in his *Hibernia Curiosa*, comparing them to Vauxhall Gardens in London.

> They have their summer entertainments too in imitation of those in London. Adjoining the Lying-in Hospital above mentioned, and belonging to it, is a large square piece of ground enclosed, and three sides out of four prettily laid out in walks and plantations of groves, shrubs, trees, etc. On the fourth stands the hospital. In the middle, nearly, of the garden is a spacious and beautiful bowling green. On the

side of the garden opposite the hospital the ground being much higher is formed into a fine hanging bank of nearly 30ft slope on top of which is laid out a grand terrace walk commanding a fine view of the hospital. On the upper side of the terrace and nearly encompassed with the groves and shrubberies is built a very pretty orchestra. This is the most agreeable garden about Dublin and is their Vauxhall. And though the whole garden is not so generally calculated for a music entertainment as the gardens of Vauxhall yet there are some walks in it where the music has a finer effect than I ever found in the London Vauxhall.

(Bush, 1764)

Vauxhall Gardens were opened in 1660 on the south bank of the River Thames up-stream from the city. Another garden in London, called Ranelagh, opened in 1742, a date which corresponded to a visit to England by Mosse, ostensibly 'to perfect himself in surgery and midwifery' (Wilde, 1846, p. 568). Ranelagh perhaps provides the clearest precedent for Dublin's New Pleasure Gardens. There, a scenic backdrop was provided by a classically inspired institutional building, the Chelsea Hospital, which, like the Royal Hospital in Dublin, was a retirement home for ex-soldiers. Clothed in their scarlet garb, the pensioners may have been called upon occasionally to enhance the spectacle of the gardens. Unlike Dublin, at Ranelagh the hospital had arrived first. The foundation stone was laid in 1681 by Charles II with the building work extending over the following decade. The architecture and dimensions of the hospital provided the organising principle for the 'constructions and plantings' of the gardens (Stevenson, 2000, p. 58; Figure 21).

In Dublin, Sackville Mall and the New Pleasure Gardens together, formed a sequence of spaces dedicated to conspicuous display and spectacle. The pleasure gardens quickly became a vortex of fashion, where parading the latest costumes accompanied evenings spent eating, drinking and promenading the gravel walks which snaked through its plantations and groves. All was accompanied by the very best and latest in fashionable music. Unlike its aristocratic sibling, the house and gardens at Kildare House, where admission was dependent upon the earl's favours or an eminent position in the social hierarchy, at Mosse's pleasure gardens freedom of entrance was based on ability to pay. Luxury and leisure were beginning to seep beyond the exclusive domain of the aristocracy and into a more (if still limited) public realm. For the price of the admission fee, the upwardly mobile could echo Mosse's achievements; mingle with the elite, ape their habits and assume temporary possession of their

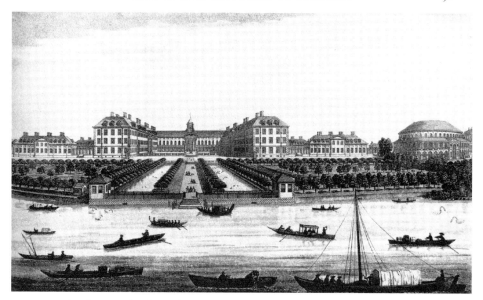

21 Royal Hospital and Ranelagh Gardens, London. (Thomas Bowles, London, 1744.)

environment. This commercial nature, however, also meant competition from other venues. In London, throughout the second half of the eighteenth century Vauxhall and Ranelagh vied with each other to be the city's 'most luxuriant resort' (Porter, 1994, p. 174). This manifested itself in a race to produce more novel and exotic phenomena than the other to titillate and entice more visitors (Ogborn, 1998, pp 116–29). The production of the fantastic, the illusory and the luxurious became an economic necessity as the landscape of amusements cultivated within the demesne accelerated into a landscape of attractions. A similar pattern of competition emerged between Dublin's various musical venues with a constant turnover of new gimmicks being offered by astute showmen as well as the almost perpetually offered performances of works 'for this first time in this Kingdom' (Boydell, 1988, p. 13). These venues included open air spaces such as St Stephen's Green, the City Bason in James' Street (Figure 22) and, not far from the southern limit of Sackville Mall, Marlborough Bowling Green (Figure 23).

To this list we can also add Ranelagh Garden's Dublin namesake, laid-out to the south-east of the city (in the present day suburb of Ranelagh) which opened in 1766. Each of these was in direct competition with Mosse. The ever-increasing search for the new, the peculiar and the idiosyncratic, not only influenced the lists of musical and theatrical entertainments, but also began to impact on the design of the landscape and other built installations within

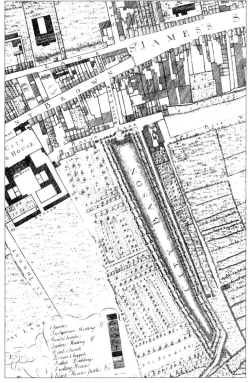

22 City Bason. (John Rocque, *Exact Survey*, 1757.)

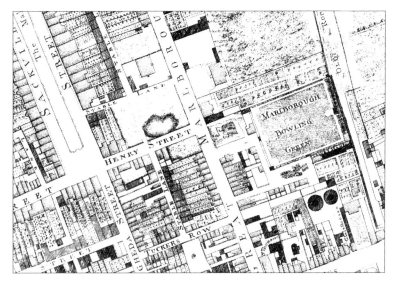

23 Marlborough Bowling Green. Note its proximity to the southern end of Sackville Street. (John Rocque, *Exact Survey*, 1756.)

Mosse's New Pleasure Gardens. In 1763, for example, the orchestra was replaced by a much more elaborate one, designed by Simon Vierpyl, for £299 11s. The hospital's records contain other, tantalising glimpses:

> 1748–1750, 'receipts for trees'
>
> 1763, payments including those for the construction of the 'new orchestra'.
>
> 22 May 1775, invoice for 'ironwork on waterfall.'
>
> 25 May 1775, receipt for 'bird to fly across waterfall.'
>
> 1775, invoice for 'work done on Gardens including Pluto's Palace.'
>
> [n.d.] receipt for carpenters' work in Garden, 'taking down temple and putting it up again.'
>
> (RHR)

While behind the façade of the hospital, medical science was attempting to produce a rational, ordered and unambiguous account of the body, the pleasure gardens were the site of so many illusions, a dream-world where nothing was quite as it seemed. Like the eighteenth-century demesne, the gardens' finite space necessitated formal devices to create the appearance of spaciousness. Landscape features beyond its boundary walls were visually framed and given context within the gardens' immediate landscape, distorting perceptions of near and far or inside and outside. The demands of novelty required a rapid turnover of phenomena. The 'waterfall' cited above proved to be mere illusion, a device which required no major earthworks and could be dismantled as rapidly as it was erected. Moreover, it had none of the drawbacks of the real: no damp, muddy pathways or the risk of splashes damaging fine dresses or worse, landing on ladies' skin.

> In the upper Walk of the Garden, above the Illuminated Temple, will be exhibited fine View of a Satyr's Cave (painted by Mr Bamford) which changes to a beautiful Representation of Water-fall; it will be shewn between the second and third Acts of the concert, for the Space of ten Minutes only. There will be Wind Music in the Garden during the Exhibition; and it is particularly requested that no Person will attempt to force the Ballustrade.
>
> (*Hibernian Journal*, 12–15 May 1775)

Such ephemeral interventions were by far the most numerous. Fireworks were often used in the intervals between musical performances as well as for spectaculars usually to commemorate some military victory or other patriotic event. On 11 September 1749, for example, Handel's *Music for the Royal Fireworks*, was performed to celebrate the peace of Aix-la-Chappelle at one of the rival venues, Marlborough Bowling Green. Competition also necessitated wider publicity. Details of forthcoming spectacles and high-profile performers were advertized in the relatively new phenomenon of newspapers, a flurry of which were founded in Dublin in the eighteenth century. In July 1772, one such publication, the *Hibernian Journal*, stated that the pleasure gardens would be illuminated and accompanied by 'a magnificent Set of Fireworks', in celebration of the anniversary of the Battle of Aughrim on 15 July. The illumination of the gardens, however, was often extended to the architecture of the hospital; in 1761, for example, an invoice was sent to the governors for 'illuminating the Lying-in Hospital for the King's marriage and coronation' (RHR). As has been shown, Mosse also engaged in singular gestures of largesse such as free breakfasts. Mrs Delany, the contemporary diarist, described one such event at the hospital, highlighting its popularity, but also, pointedly, its mixed company. The room she describes is the 'Long Room' located on the western edge of the garden and shown on Rocque's *Exact Survey*. Her 'job-description' of Mosse is also very interesting, making no reference to either midwifery, surgery or medicine.

> Delville, February 1750–51 – Dr Moss you must know is the chief manager and operator of the Lying-in Hospital, and has gardens laid out in the manner of Vauxhall and Ranelagh; and in order to gather together subscribers for the next season he gave a gratis breakfast and a fine concert of music in a large room which was not opened before, and is in the gardens. The music allured us, and, we went, D.D. [Dr Delaney, the dean of Down] with us, at about half an hour after eleven, the concert to begin at 12. When we came, with some difficulty we squeezed into the room, which they say is 60ft long, and got up to the breakfast table, which had been well pillaged; the fragments of cakes, bread and butter, silver coffee-pots, and tea kettles without number, and all sorts of spring flowers strewn on the table, shewed it had been set out plentifully and elegantly. The company, indeed, looked as if their principal design of coming was for a breakfast. When they had

satisfied their hunger the remains were taken away, and such a rude mob (for they deserved no better name) crowded in that I and my company crowded out as fast as we could, glad to escape in whole skins, and resolving never more to add to the throng of a gratis entertainment.
(Delany, in Llanover, 1926, p. 185)

It has been suggested Mosse's gardens were the finest on the city: neither, 'James' Street Basin nor the promenading of St Stephen's Green, which Swift recommended to Stella as superior to the London Mall, offered anything to the inducements held out by Dr Mosse to the citizens' (Curran, 1947, p. 29). In comparison, Marlborough Bowling Green was a flat square of land and St Stephen's Green was a vast space divided into four and bounded at its edges by a rather monotonous, regimented and uniform row of trees. The City Bason could offer the allure of a body of water, especially potent for the display of fireworks, but little in the way of spaces in which to gather or a diversity of walks. Bush's description (above) of the New Pleasure Gardens, on the other hand, suggested an integrated relationship between music, scenery and architecture, where each part influenced and reinforced the effect of the others. The centrality of the orchestra meant music could penetrate unseen into the remotest nooks and corners of the garden. The terrace, moreover, was perfectly situated to appreciate the façade of the hospital as well as the activities of the bowling green while the meandering walks offered unexpected vistas and views. Ranelagh Gardens may have been a stronger rival. Its grounds were laid out with the benefit of the Mosse's pleasure gardens as a prototype and its owner, William Holister was similarly disposed to spectacular interventions in the landscape, arranging, for example, for the road from the city to his suburban site to be illuminated on musical nights. He also occasionally presented 'tumblers, rope-dancers and balloon ascents' (Boydell, 1992, p. 21). His enterprise, however, closed down due to bankruptcy only nine years after it opened.

Only the New Pleasure Gardens had the potent combination of architecture, aristocratic patronage and charity as permanent features. Indeed, despite the obvious debts to London's Vauxhall and the influence of competition and commercialism, the New Pleasure Gardens' qualities as a landscape of spectacle and amusement can never be completely divorced from its relationship with charity. Some of the most profitable concerts in the city were those given for the benefit of charitable foundations (Boydell, 1992, p. 21). At the New Pleasure Gardens, visitors were constantly reminded of where their admission fees and refreshment expenses were destined, by the 'fine views of

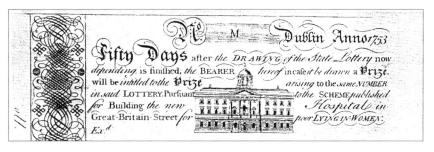

24 Lottery ticket displaying the Lying-in Hospital elevation, 1753. (RHR)

the hospital'. The building's Palladian front façade became a form of advertising, the motif disseminated on a variety of printed media; lottery tickets (Figure 24), admission tickets, even Mosse's personal notepaper. The hospital represented charity in a most immediate and tangible form. Moreover, it was magnificent. It simultaneously satisfied an ethos which stated that 'in comparison of things that are good, the largest, the most publick, the most lasting ought to have pre-eminence' (Stillingfleet, 1681, quoted in Campbell-Ross, ed., 1986, p. 17), as well as the demands of a discerning set of consumers for an elaborate backdrop for their entertainments.

The presence of aristocracy, especially the lord lieutenant, also added immeasurably to the popularity of any concert or evening's entertainment. The pleasure gardens and Lying-in Hospital, complete with Royal Charter and aristocratic governors enjoyed the patronage and seal of approval from the country's elite. As charity merged seamlessly into spectacle and vice-versa, both bore the identity and ethos of their sponsors.

The separated spheres of labour and leisure

The suggestion that the demesne was a type of utopia implies a landscape of order and harmony in which an apparent spirit of mutual consent between the varied social strata of the household's members contributed to its ongoing success and productivity (O'Kane, 2000). In this landscape everything and everyone was compelled to know its place and conform to a given hierarchy. This was reflected in a finely-tuned differentiation of space – an understood and accepted code which distinguished between served and serving spaces as well as navigating the nuanced transitions from public to private zones. Decoration was central to this code. Sumptuous public rooms displayed the family's wealth through elaborate furnishings and the delicate hand of the

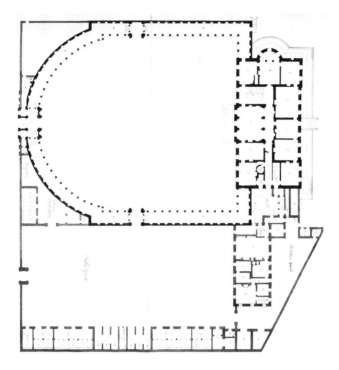

25 Kildare House, ground floor plan and courtyard. Note the *enfilade* arrangement of the rooms of the garden front (right hand-side) of the house. (Richard Cassels, *c.*1745.)

stuccodore while spaces of utility and labour, unadorned and prosaic, lay concealed behind screens or occupied non central areas such as side wings, basements or attics. Servants and workers were similarly disposed; 'hands' whose labour sustained the house either faded into invisibility or else, suitably attired, became part of the decor.

At Kildare House, the grand entrance courtyard which addressed the front façade was paralleled by a stable-yard (Figure 25). Separated by a screen wall, the latter was also served by its own discrete entrance and contained the kitchens, servants' accommodation and many of the house's other necessities. Within the main block other services were contained in the basement. On the other hand, the ground and first floors, linked by the main stairs, hosted a series of grand public rooms where guests could be entertained. These two principal floors, however, also contained private apartments where members of the family could retire when not receiving visitors. As well as the double-height entrance hall, the ground floor contained a private dining area. The first floor or *piano nobile* contained the earl and countess's bedrooms and

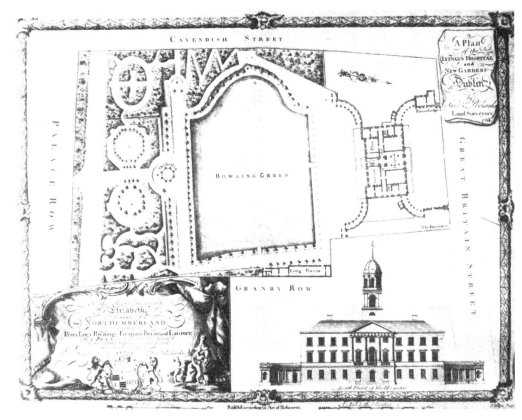

26 The new Lying-in Hospital and gardens (Sarlé and Richards, 1764, drawings dedicated to Elizabeth, duchess of Northumberland). The modest patients' entrance is located off the top right colonnade. The colonnaded wings to the garden side have been added since 1757 (compare with Figure 17 above). Note also that the *enfilade* arrangement on the ground floor plan of Kildare House is not repeated in the Hospital where the sequence of rooms along the garden front is broken by the central staircase.

private drawing room as well as the huge double height-gallery. The second floor or attic storey was less well appointed. In other villas it was often used for servants' accommodation. In Kildare House, however, it was occupied by the children's bedrooms and nursery, reflecting a contemporary attitude which often placed children only slightly above servants in the household hierarchy.

Notwithstanding obvious differences in function, the Lying-in Hospital contained a similar spatial hierarchy. While the commercial pleasure gardens allowed some mixing of different social classes, admission was still limited to the small section of society who could afford the entrance fee. In 1772, sixpence was paid for broken bottles for the top of the garden wall to stop people climbing over ('Draft of Miscellaneous Account Book 1772', RHR) while at Vauxhall, a device called the 'coop' spared visitors the sight of groups of loitering servants awaiting their masters' return (Ogborn, 1998, p. 120). Entrance to the New Pleasure Gardens was from Great-Britain Street, just beyond the edge of the western colonnade, where visitors would present their tickets or pay their money. The space wedged behind this colonnade and its garden counterpart may have been used in a similar way to dispose of servants. The hospital's central doorway was used by 'officers' such as Mosse and for the chapel on Sundays. Pregnant women seeking admission to the hospital or their visitors, however, experienced an entirely different sequence of access. They entered on the eastern side of the building through an unassuming door in the colonnade. From there they turned left through a side door to where the Registrar's Office was located. Immediately adjacent was the eastern 'back stairs', allowing rapid and unseen access to the wards above (Figure 26).

Patients' admission was, in fact, a fairly complicated process involving more than one trip to the hospital and a set timetable.

> [T]he Patient must attend at the Hospital on Monday, Wednesday, or Friday, between the hours of Ten and Twelve in the Forenoon, with her Certificate, which (if approved of) is to be signed by the Master of the Hospital, or by such Person as he shall appoint. And such Certificate, so signed shall entitle the Owner thereof, or the Person thereby recommended, to be received into the Hospital, when she comes to her Time of Lying-in (provided she submit to the Rules of the House).
> ('Entry Certificate', 1759, RHR)

According to the hospital's rules printed on the admission certificate, visiting hours were limited to between 10 a.m. and 12 noon By 1769, however, Sundays and Public Holidays were excluded. The following extract from Faulkner's *Dublin Journal* perhaps reveals why, detailing some of the disorder which could accompany visits by working-class spouses.

> Lying-in Hospital, January 4th, 1769 – Whereas many melancholy Accidents have happened in said Hospital, by Patients drinking intoxicating liquors privately brought in by their friends, who are permitted to visit them (Sundays and Public Holidays excepted)

between the Hours of Ten and Twelve. The Master of said Hospital thinks it necessary to give in Public Notice, that for the Future no Person whatsoever will be permitted to visit the patients who will not submit to be searched at the gate. And requests that Ladies will not desire to send Wines or any Provisions to their Servants who may be Patients as everything proper and requisite for them is allowed at the expense of the Hospital.

(Faulkner's *Dublin Journal*, 5, 7 and 10 January 1769)

On Sundays the chapel was used for fund-raising sermons. Public holidays in the gardens were likely to be amongst the busiest days of the year often boasting additional entertainments. Both were crucial to the economic viability of the institution. Unsolicited images of groups of ill-clad husbands loitering about, or worse drunken (expectant) mothers having 'melancholy accidents' would have perhaps represented an affront to the harmony of such occasions. In fact, as shall be shown, it was not necessarily the patients or their relatives who were the main perpetrators of such disturbances.

Internally, the adaptation of the model of a large villa to form the Lying-in Hospital required no major changes: a similar pattern of spatial segregation applied. A full set of plans and sections of the hospital, produced in 1788 for the marquis of Buckingham, shows the layout and functions of the different rooms. Like Kildare House the basement of the Lying-in Hospital contained services: kitchens, pantries, stores and a laundry. The ground floor contained at its centre the main entrance hall which led to the great staircase after crossing the central corridor which, like at Kildare House, bisected the building longitudinally. On the southern, street-side, to the east of the entrance were the 'Chaplains' Apartments' forming an L-shape around the small 'Registrar's Office'. To the west were the 'Pupils Apartments' for medical students, followed by the 'House Surgeon's Apartment' on the south-western corner. From west to east on the northern, garden-side was the Matron's Apartment, followed by the Board Room. Beyond the main stairs was the Master's Apartment which Mosse occupied until his death. The main stair served the 'Ground Floor' and 'Principal [first] Floor' only. Two other 'back' staircases, one at either end, served the rest of the building. By 1788, the northern side of the 'Principal Floor' was entirely occupied by ward space; two large and four smaller ones. Wards, however, were entirely absent from the southern side. Instead, its centre was taken up by three public rooms; the double storey 'Chapel' flanked on its west and east side by the 'Anti-Chapel'

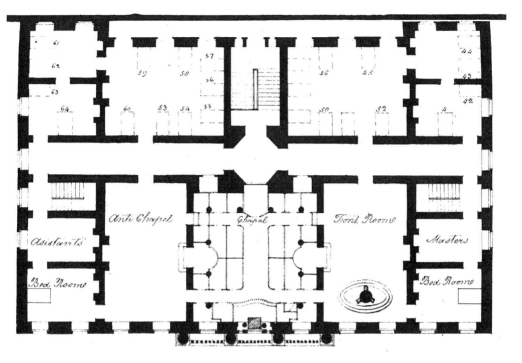

27 Plan of the 'Principal Floor' of the Lying-in Hospital. Note the arrangement of the pews which are mainly orientated perpendicular to the altar.
(Drawn for the marquis of Buckingham, 1788.)

and the 'Font Room' respectively. At either end of the block the Master's and Assistants Bedrooms completed the floor (Figure 27).

The attic storey, or 'Bed-chamber Floor', 'furnished with fifty beds and all other requisites', was finished before the rest of the hospital in 1757 (Wilde, 1846, p. 581) (see appendix 2: extracts from the Lying-in Hospital Account Book, 1757). In fact, the number of beds did not increase between 1759 and 1763, after the chapel had been finished. During these years the wards were confined solely to the attic storey, the equivalent of the children's space at Kildare House. There was, however, one exception. The 'Upper part of Chapel' contained a small wooden U-shaped gallery, accessed from the central corridor, which looked down into the chapel proper below. Unlike Kildare House, the *piano nobile* and the attic storey shared a space (Figures 28 and 29).

The opening ceremony in 1757 was symptomatic of the intersection between spectacle and charity at the hospital and its tactful negotiation between display and concealment. Attended by the lord lieutenant, the duke

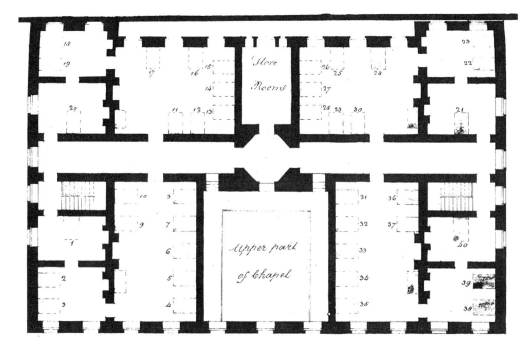

28 Plan of 'Bed-chamber Floor' of Lying-in Hospital. The 'Upper Part of Chapel' is bounded on three sides by the wooden (inverted) U-shaped gallery. (Drawn for the marquis of Buckingham, 1788.)

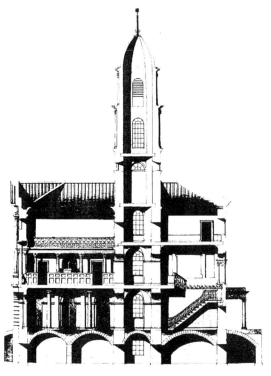

29 Cross-section of Lying-in Hospital. Note the double-height chapel and women's gallery with elaborate balustrade. (Drawn for the marquis of Buckingham, 1788.)

of Bedford, his wife and a gaggle of aristocracy, it was significant because it represented the first moment of interface between two groups at either end of the social scale: the hospital's benefactors and its beneficiaries. When the gardens opened in 1748, the lying-in patients had been only a distant reality, sequestered in George's Lane, safely out of sight of the pleasure-seeking crowds. As Wilde's biographical note of Mosse suggests, upper-class connections to 'charitable objects' tended to be moderated, and conditions of poverty concealed within the city fabric.

> In the course of [Mosse's] practice charity demanded his assistance; and he hath often declared that the misery of the poor women of the city of Dublin, at the time of their lying-in would scarcely be conceived by anyone who had not been an eye witness of their wretched circumstances.
> (Wilde, 1846, p. 568)

At the ceremony, Mosse tempered the potential shock of proximity by appealing to the established convention of the site: he put the women on display as part of the spectacle.

> [F]ifty-two women great with child attended in the hall with proper certificates for admission, and were all decently clothed in uniform at the expense of the hospital, each in a blue calimanco gown and petticoat, shift, handkerchief, cap and apron and thus appeared before His Grace as President of the Hospital, the Duchess, and the rest of the Governors and Guardians, with many of the nobility and gentry, who all expressed the highest satisfaction. During the whole time of breakfast and the ceremony of opening the hospital, their Graces and the company were entertained by a concert, of vocal and instrumental music, and everything was conducted in the most regular, easy and genteel manner.
> (Wilde, 1846, p. 581)

The encounter was formal and prescribed. They met each other in the quietly opulent surroundings of the main hall at the front of the building (Figure 30). The women, sartorially altered to fit the occasion, had a pleasingly colourful veneer, but perhaps more importantly, a uniformity which made them conform to an image of deserving objects of charity; clean, ordered and mostly indistinguishable. Moreover, they were not a representative cross-section of the city's pregnant population.

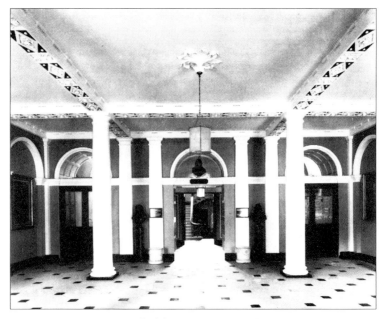

30 Entrance Hall of the Lying-in Hospital. (Casey, 1986.)

Entry to the Lying-in Hospital was conditional to the fulfilment of strict requirements. Until 1780, when the right was extended to the Catholic priesthood, good character had to be pledged by a member of the Established clergy in a form addressed to Mosse, the Master of the Hospital.

> Sir, We the Minister and Church-wardens of the Parish of _____ recommend _____ as a proper Object; and if upon Examination she shall appear such to you, desire she may be received into the Hospital.

The regulations also stipulated that the women had to be free from certain disorders:

> That no Woman great with Child is to be received into the Hospital if she hath any Contagious Distemper, or the Venereal Disease.
> ('Entry Certificate', 1750s, RHR)

After the women had been presented and inspected, the visitors moved on into the pleasure gardens or to the Coffee Room where further entertainments awaited. The patients, on the other hand, took the back stairs to the wards at the top of the house. Later that day, one or two of them would give birth; a midwife fumbling with an incoming life, unseen by the mêlée below. The costs for the opening were £167 17s. 27d. (see appendix: extracts from the Lying-in Hospital Account Book, 1757). A total of £182 18s. 2½d. was collected in donations from the invited guests.

Protestantism and productivity

In 1755, Mosse made the first of a number of appeals to Parliament for additional funds to construct the hospital. In March 1756 he was granted £6,000. In 1757, he appealed once more to complete the building. This time the hospital was awarded £6,000 and Mosse himself, £2,000:

> [A]s a Reward for his great Care and Diligence in attending the Lying-in Hospital in George's Lane, thirteen Years, and superintending the new Hospital in Great-Britain-street nine Years and an Half, by which he hath greatly injured himself in his Profession, and hurt his Family in their Circumstance, having never received any Reward.
> (*Journals of the Irish House of Commons*, 6 and 23 March 1756)

After Mosse's death, the governors met to discuss the state of the hospital and found it was in debt. Following another application, Parliament awarded £3,000 to the hospital and a further £1,000 to Mrs Mosse. There were similar petitions in November 1761 and November 1763, resulting in an additional payment of £3,000 to the hospital and £1,000 to Mrs Mosse (Wilde, 1846, pp 592–3). The hospital's consistent success in obtaining Parliamentary funds suggests an intersection of interests. No other voluntary hospital in the city achieved the same level of Parliamentary funding. In comparison, St Patrick's, Ireland's first mental hospital, received only £1,000 in 1756 from Parliament and its opening passed off without any ceremony at all which suggests that there was significantly less enthusiasm for 'Swift's gloomy madhouse on Bow Lane' (Malcolm, 1989, p. 37), despite a decent sprinkling of clergy and gentry on its board of governors.

Equally, as evinced by the lists published in Watson's *Almanack*, no other hospital boasted a board of governors strewn with so many members of both the Commons and the Lords as the Lying-in. The limited electoral franchise – Catholics were not allowed to vote or sit in Parliament – meant that, almost to a man, these members were land-owning Protestants. As a site where culture was produced and disseminated, patrons of the hospital and gardens were able to bask in a self-reflecting celebration of the magnificent achievements of Irish Protestantism. This underlying meaning was insinuated everywhere; in the everyday culture of manners, in the music, in the architecture and landscape, as well as more explicit proclamations like the spectacles commemorating significant moments in the recent victorious history of Protestant Ireland. Individual representatives of the Anglo-Irish class, however, were also singled out.

In 1757, Mosse commissioned John van Nost to produce a series of sculptures for the gardens. These were mostly inspired by mythical figures from antiquity: Antonious, Venus de Medici, Mercury, Apollo, Janus and a sitting Venus. Mosse 'also intended erecting a magnificent statue of Juno Lucina (the heathen goddess presiding over women in labour), and to call the garden Lucinda's Garden' (Wilde, 1846, p. 583). Into this pantheon of deities, Mosse inserted some of his longest standing supporters, commissioning marble busts of Lord Sudley (Sir Arthur Gore), Lord Shannon and the bishop of Clogher. Another was scheduled to be a likeness of Kildare, but the earl apparently refused to sit for it, perhaps reasoning that his identity at the hospital was already well-represented. Van Nost was also commissioned to 'execute two large statues in lead and to be bronzed in gold' of George II and the prince of Wales for the two niches at the end of the front-colonnades (Wilde, 1846, p. 584). Amongst the ideological possibilities, however, charity was perhaps the most powerful. The various inflections of the word used in the eighteenth century include, '[t]he Christian love of our fellow-men; Christian benignity of disposition expressing itself in Christ-like conduct'. To bestow charity was to assume a powerful position which had historical as well as contemporary connotations.

At the Lying-in Hospital, the fusion of charity, spectacle and religious significance was at its most powerful in the dream-like space of the chapel. Finished in 1762, behind the building's prosaic façade lay the unexpected jewel in the landscape of attractions: a baroque extravaganza which Mosse 'intended should excel anything of that size in Europe' (Wilde, 1846, p. 585). Located at the centre front of the *piano nobile*, it occupied a prime position in the building's composition. In elevation, its area, beginning above the rusticated ground floor, is both enclosed within and announced by the Doric temple-front motif (Figure 31). This differs from Kildare House where the temple-front is shared by two discrete spaces; the double-height entrance hall and the central rooms of the attic storey. Two pedimented windows flank a Palladian window on the first floor, above which, on the second floor, the central window is shortened, while the two side windows follow the same proportions as the rest of the elevation. This arrangement, which perhaps hints at the

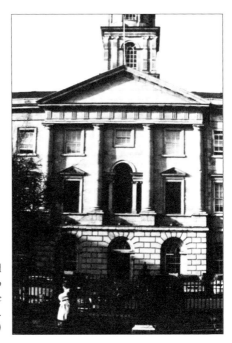

31 The vertical columns, entablature and triangular pediment which make up the classical temple front exhibited here on the Lying-in Hospital's front façade. (Author's photograph.)

double height within, appears to have been perceived as a mistake on the part of Cassels. Subsequently, almost every architect, draughtsman or artist to make a representation of the façade, has taken pains to perfect it, by making the side windows the same dimensions as the centre one (see, for example, the renderings of the building's façade in Figures 26).

The chapel was approached through a sequence of well-appointed spaces, whose decoration directed the gaze and delineated a processional route. Visitors entered the stone flagged entrance hall of the hospital through the central door. From there, they moved through the centre arch of three into the main stairs. Here, the gaze was focused upwards by the plaster 'foliar motifs' of Robert West and the large Palladian window at the half-landing (Casey in Campbell-Ross, ed., 1986, p. 58). This window allowed the visitor to catch a panorama of the gardens before returning upwards. At the top of the stairs, entry to the chapel was either directly from the landing or else via the 'Anti-Chapel' or the 'Font-Room' located at either side and described collectively in the Hospital Minutes of 1 February 1782, as 'rooms of parade'. Once inside, the proportions of the chapel, a square 36 x 36ft and 30ft high, threw the gaze upwards where it rested upon 'a ceiling without parallel in Ireland, ... a full-bloodied baroque treatment with figures in whole relief, cherubs, terms, bunches of grapes and ribbands of text flying out from the cove' (Craig, 1992, p. 144). The introspective quality of the space was enhanced by a lack of visual connection to the outside. The Palladian window and its two flanking windows were of stained glass. Moreover, the three upper windows, visible from the outside, fail to make an appearance at all in the interior, exposing the disjunction between the compositional requirements of the elevation and the interior space. The central window has completely vanished behind a plaster figure, while those to either side are obscured by an ingenious set of shutters which continue both the wall plane and the cornice moulding and allow some control over the natural light entering the space. The ceiling was intended to be even more elaborate. Mosse's death in February 1759 terminated plans for a Mr Cipriani, a painter living in London, to execute a series of five biblical parables in its central panel and the four attached cartouches. A series of letters between the two, dating from 1758 and extensively quoted by Wilde, demonstrate the extent of Mosse's involvement in the scheme. Appropriately, he chose narratives concerning childbirth and midwifery. He also, however, explained his decisions by reference to the stories' expressive possibilities. In a choice between the Nativity and the Ascension, for example, '[m]y inclination tends rather to the Nativity, as more susceptible of poetical images'. Similarly, the fury of Pharaoh when he discovered the midwives had not carried out his wishes to kill newborn males seemed to afford full scope for the genius of the painter to exercise himself, Mosse, however, also pointedly reminded Cipriani of the hospital and chapel's religious affiliations.

> As this chapel is intended only for Protestant worship, I would have the painting entirely free from any superstitious or Popish representation.

To which Cipriani replied, in a postscript,

> I forgot to tell you that you shall have no other Popery in the picture than the Nativity of Our Saviour; and, as I am pretty sure that the Pope shall never set foot in Ireland, so you may be confident that my picture will never contribute to the enlargement of His Holiness's jurisdiction.
> (quoted in Wilde, 1846, pp 588–9)

Meanwhile, Cramillion the stuccodore, had created three principal figures, female incarnations of the Pauline virtues: Faith, Hope and Charity. High in an alcove on the east wall, Faith is blindfolded, holding a cross and a plummet and is treading on a fox which overhangs the cornice. Opposite, on the west wall, Hope is holding an anchor. On the south wall, Charity, in the guise of a young mother, suckles an infant with two young children playing around her

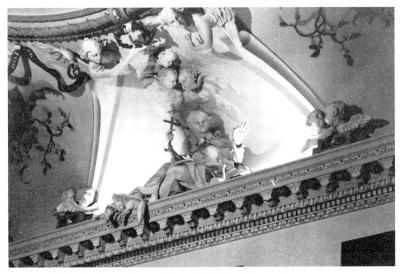

32 Lying-in Hospital chapel. Detail: Faith holding a plummet and cross. (Author's photograph.)

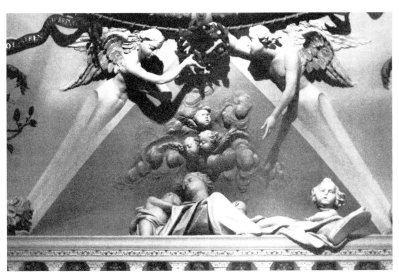

33 Lying-in Hospital chapel. Detail: Charity. The plaster figure hides the central window which can be seen on the external elevation. (Author's photograph.)

(Figures 32 and 33). Her form and privileged position immediately above the altar, (the hidden central window is behind her) underpins the importance of charity both in the hospital's ethos and contemporary Protestant society where, 'now abideth faith, hope and charity, these three and the greatest of these is charity' (1 Corinthians 13:13).

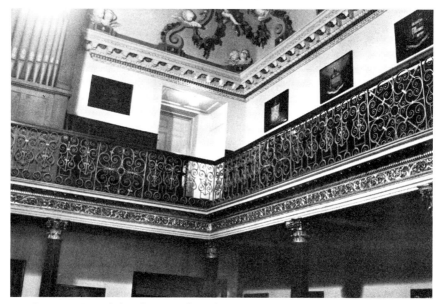

34 Lying-in Hospital chapel interior, from the 'Principal Floor' showing balcony where the pregnant women sat and its relationship to the ceiling. (Author's photograph.)

As the patrons' gaze was directed from their mahogany pews heavenwards towards the ceiling it also, however, caught sight of the real lying-in women on the upper gallery. Through the gauze-like iron railings visitors could just perceive swollen bodies and nodding heads and perhaps hear, in the pauses between the preacher's expostulations and the baroque notes of the organist, the intermittent rustle of clothing (Figure 34).

The chapel, stretching between the *piano nobile* and the attic storey was a moment of connection between the patients and their benefactors. Like the opening ceremony, however, the encounter was highly prescribed. The women were viewed against a backdrop of representations of perfect virtue and morality. The significance of the chapel and its relationship with the hospital is perhaps best revealed in a sermon written in 1759 by a Reverend Lawson to celebrate its opening. It began with a quotation from the Bible,

> They shall bring thy Sons in their Arms, and Daughters shall be carried on their Shoulders
>
> (Isaiah 49:22)

He explained the significance of the words and their contemporary appropriateness.

These words are part of a magnificent Description, which the Prophet gives of the future conversion of the Gentiles, and their final union with the church of Christ. And they paint the Proselytes to this Religion as Being called out of a State of Slavery and Ignorance, into Liberty and Light, crowding to embrace this heavenly Doctrine, and marching in a kind of triumphal Procession. These Expressions are thus applied by the Prophet in a figurative sense, to celebrate this great Event permit me to employ in their literal signification, to recommend a principal Duty, the distinguishing characteristick of this Holy Religion, Charity; an excellent Branch whereof ye meet this Day to consider, and are noticed to encourage. Ye easily see that the words in their plainest direct sense present to your Eyes a lively Image of the Effect which your Liberality here tends to produce; 'Disconsolate Women going from hence joyful Mothers'.

(Lawson, 1759)

Lawson's choice of this excerpt concerning conversion and the positive aspects of proselytizing is suggestive of the significance of the chapel and, indeed the hospital, in eighteenth-century Ireland. While the initial register from 1745 (Figure 65) does not record religious affiliation, perhaps because the patients were generally Protestant, later registers (Figure 66) record that the majority of women who gave birth there were Catholics (or 'Papists'). The centrality of the chapel and its connection with the attic storey meant its presence and meaning could pervade all the wards; the Protestant ethos present at the very moment of creation. Furthermore, it was proposed that a Protestant Chaplain, would 'baptize all the Children, Church the women [a rite of purification given after child-birth, only after which could they enter the church and receive the sacrament] and punctually discharge all the other Clerical duties of the said Hospital' ('Doctor King, chaplain setting down duties' (undated), RHR). Mosse also proposed a scheme where female midwives from all Ireland's counties would be sent to Dublin to train at the hospital, as a 'means of preventing the unhappy effects owing to the ignorance of the generality of country midwives' (*Royal Charter*, 1756). This also meant, however, that throughout the country wherever life sprung into existence, it would be guided into the world by a hand trained at the Protestant hospital. Indeed, in his sermon Lawson soon turned his attention to the hospital's productive possibilities, which he expressed in terms of 'public utility'. Addressing the congregation as 'Christians, Citizens and Men', he described the benefit of their charity to 'our Creator, our Country, and Human Nature,' making it clear that the hospital and its chapel were at the heart of a wider strategy.

> For the chief Foundation of the Prosperity of a State is, the Multitude of Inhabitants; it grows usually in Wealth and Power as it becomes Populous. For this reason the wisest states have always applied themselves with much attention to procure and encrease the Number of their People ... Now the Tendency of the Charitable Foundation this Day before us, to produce this national Effect is manifest. I need not say how large a Proportion of the unhappy Mothers or wretched Infants preserved here must have otherwise perished; it is certainly not inconsiderable. If then you suppose this scheme executed to its whole Extent: (a hope for the good spirit prevailing among us is likely to be fulfilled), you see that it will add no small Number of Souls to the Community; and if it had existed many Years past we should not feel in so great a Degree the present Evils arising from fewness of inhabitants ... For it has been remarked that the Encrease of Inhabitants most to be desired is among the lowest Ranks; those of Condition, or such as affect to live like those of Condition above Labour, being perhaps numerous enough: Now the direct Influence of this Charity is this Encrease; to supply Hands for Tillage, the most fertile Parts of our Island lying yet, uncultivated: For the carrying-on of Manufactures: For doing the laborious Part and Drudgery of Mechanics: For the extending of Commerce: for Maintaining the Safety and Glory of the Nation in the War-like Forces of Both Elements, sometimes at present filled up not without Difficulty. This is the Strength of a Country, the Foundation, which tho' laid into Dust, tho' rugged and obscure, do yet support whatever is raised above of polished and splendid. We have cause therefore to say that in supporting this scheme we contribute to the National Advantage, we act the Part of good Citizens, and deserve the amiable Character of Lovers of our Country.
>
> (Lawson, 1759)

The sociologist Max Weber famously suggested that the concerns of Protestantism tended to resonate closely with those of the emerging capitalist mode of production (Weber, 1930). Key Protestant values concerning the work ethic, timekeeping and respect for property, gave the new social relations of wage labour a religious justification and helped to create a new class of acquiescent workers. Weber's theories on religion, therefore, converge with Foucault's explanation of the sudden importance assumed by medicine in the eighteenth century. According to Foucault, the medical sciences during this period became intricately connected to the preservation, upkeep and conservation of the 'labour force', where the biological traits of a population became relevant factors for economic management. Moreover, he suggests that it became necessary to organize around the working classes a series of apparatuses which would ensure not only their subjection but the constant increase of their utility (Foucault, 1991, p. 278). Dublin's Lying-in Hospital seems to reflect those trends. According to the Reverend Lawson, the vision Mosse had for his hospital extended beyond childbirth and into the formation, or, as Foucault terms it, the 'correct management' of children's character.

> [A] Scheme was formed to raise a Fund sufficient to defray the Expenses of Nursing, Cloathing, and general Maintenance of these Children who should be born in the Lying-in Hospital, and whom their parents should entrust to the Doctor's Care. A School was to be opened, provided with Protestant Masters in the most useful Trades and Manufactures; into this School the Children at a proper Age, were to be received; there to be instructed in the Principles of the Christian Religion, in Honesty and Industry; and to be taught some such Trade as their Genius most strongly inclined to: And it is Fact, that with a View of this Kind, he, at his own Expense had put out some Children to be nursed, who since his Death have returned. This Scheme in short extended even to providing a comfortable subsistence for the Parents.
> (Lawson, 1759)

One of Mosse's intentions as part of this scheme was to 'establish a hardware manufacture as at Birmingham in England' (Wilde, 1846, p. 582). The training received there would ensure the avoidance of producing what Lawson termed a 'Multitude without Virtue'. Finally, Lawson delineated the role of the hospital's benefactors in these schemes.

> Kings become its nursing Fathers, Queens become its Nursing Mothers: The Legislature assist in fixing and finishing it: a wider Scene is opened, and better Prospects unfold themselves. Time and industry it is hoped will render it still more useful and extensive: Farther improvements may be thought of. The Planter's Hand now points out one, and prepares to make this Plant more fruitful by lengthening out its care from Birth in part to Education, thus rendering useful the life it saveth.
> (Lawson, 1759)

A ward in the hospital, distinguished by the King's Arms, was called the Parliament Ward, another, bearing the City Arms was called the City of Dublin Ward (Campbell-Ross, in idem, 1986, p. 27). Benefactors could also

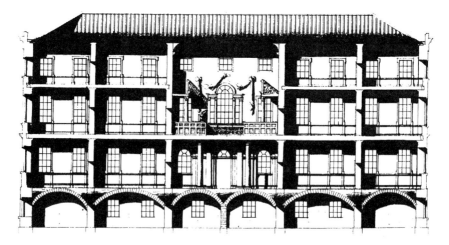

35 Long section of Lying-in Hospital. Note the double-height space of the chapel containing the women's gallery above the patrons' pews which like the relationship of the wealthy patrons' boxes to the stage at the Theatre Royal (Figure 19), are placed perpendicular to the altar (see also Figure 27). (Drawn for the marquis of Buckingham, 1788.)

sponsor beds in the hospital. Erecting a bed cost £12 15s. 9d. and running costs were £12 10s. per annum thereafter. Each bed relieved approximately sixteen women per year. The list for 1761 read: the marquis of Kildare (2 beds), earl of Kerry, Lord Viscount Charlemont, Rt Hon. Mr Gardiner, His Excellency John Ponsonby (in 1756, the Speaker of the House of Commons), Rt Hon. Mr Clements, Rt Hon. Sir William Yorke, Richard Dawson Esq., James Taylor Esq., Mr Clayton, John Putland Esq., Queen's County (1 bed each).

As a member of The Dublin Society, Mosse was familiar with the ideologies of improvement. His vision, however, called for their application to be extended firmly beyond the managed cultivation of land into the managed cultivation of a certain section of society. The Lying-in Hospital, echoing the productive meaning of the villa in the landscape, facilitated and supervised the very moment of production of a new population. The chapel, then, was perhaps the purest condensation of a version of utopia, where Enlightenment notions of the perfectible nature of the human character and society, were recast within a Protestant idiom. Even here, however, its apparently rarefied atmosphere was infused with other, less idealistic agendas and external influences. After all, the chapel, like all the other phenomena in the gardens, was part of a landscape of attractions, not only a place of worship, but also a source of making money and a site of display and theatricality (Figures 34 and 35).

The hospital and the spectacular city

The death of Mosse

After Mosse's death in 1759, his vision for the Lying-in Hospital diluted and fragmented. While the appeal to parliament by the governors, led by Leinster and Sudley whom Mosse had named as the hospital's trustees in his will, was successful in paying off the institution's substantial debt and providing assistance with the completion of the hospital and chapel, some financial difficulties remained unresolved. Consequently, not only were parts of the building still incomplete as late as 1765, but some of Mosse's more extravagant notions were abandoned. Cipriani's plan for the chapel ceiling was cancelled, Juno Lucina never graced the gardens and a new pavilion which Mosse had intended to stand on the garden's east side next to Cavendish Row came to nothing. Similarly, the statues produced by Van Nost, with the exception of the busts of the bishop of Clogher and Lord Shannon, were all returned to the sculptor. Van Nost, however, was given one final commission to produce a likeness of Mosse from his death mask (*Irish Builder*, March 1897, p. 59) and a living legacy to the hospital's founder was provided by the appointment of Mosse's nephew, the Revd Thomas Mosse as hospital chaplain. Other more significant aspects to Mosse's vision for his hospital and its place in society also remained unimplemented. His manufacturing school, designed to instruct its students, under the tutelage of Protestant masters, in the principles of 'Christian Religion, in Honesty and Industry', was never executed. Similarly, his scheme to provide nursing, clothing and maintenance to those born at the hospital was abandoned soon after his death and all the children involved were returned to their birth parents (Wilde, 1846, p. 582).

With Kildare and Sudley's role as trustees, the decision-making process of the hospital, always heavily influenced by its aristocratic patrons, slipped temporarily but resolutely out of medical and surgical hands. In 1759, Fielding Ould, Mosse's replacement as Master was appointed after a competitive process. Unlike Mosse, whose mastership had been for life, Ould's tenure was limited to seven years. Moreover, the automatic entitlement of the master to be a governor was also suspended – Watson's *Almanack* of 1761 fails to list Ould as such. Indeed, of the thirty-six named governors cited in that publication only one, a Dr Ezekial Nesbitt, was a member of either the surgical or medical professions. Nesbitt was appointed as physician to the hospital and a governor immediately after Mosse's death, but his influence can be described at best as marginal. Of the fifteen years he occupied the post, he apparently spent ten of them living in Bath. Ould's term as master from 1759 to 1766 has been described as a period of consolidation characterized by a lack of money (Campbell-Ross, 1986, p. 41). From the hospital's opening in 1757 until 1763, the number of beds remained constant at fifty-two, despite the hospital being able to accommodate three times as many. In an appeal to parliament for additional funds in 1763, the governors, after detailing the hospital's existing debts, stressed that the means to address these financial shortfalls and expand the hospital lay in increasing the quality of the gardens' entertainment facilities.

> [T]he Garden belonging to the said Hospital, which has of late produced near £400 yearly, might as your petitioners apprehend, be made of much greater advantage to the hospital by building a large room for the accommodation of the company ... [I]f they were now enabled to pay the debts contracted on account of the chapel, and to build a large room and make other improvements in the garden, the said chapel and garden might produce a yearly sum, which with the present endowments would be sufficient to support a greater number of beds than are as yet erected; and ... if they were enabled to add to their Number of beds, they might relieve a greater number of patients, and thereby render the said hospital much more extensive and useful.
>
> ('Petition to Parliament by the Governors of the Lying-in Hospital', undated manuscript, RHR)

The policy of raising money by providing firstly for the needs of spectacle and entertainment proved enduring. Every subsequent major architectural development at the hospital in the eighteenth century had the pursuit of leisure as its primary function. On 15 June 1764 the governors placed an advert inviting designs and tenders for the 'large room for the accommodation of the company'. On 11 September of the same year, John Ensor's design was accepted. He was given £300 for materials and asked to begin right away. The 'large room' was to be the Rotunda.

The arrival of Charlemont and the Rotunda

At the same time as these events were taking place, other developments were happening in the hospital's vicinity. The popularity of the New Pleasure Gardens had ensured the 'very stones of Dublin began to cluster around Mosse's enterprise' (Curran, 1947, p. 29). Cavendish Row, the earliest of the gardens' adjacent streets dates from 1753 and was divided into residential plots by Mosse himself and then leased. The area's growing reputation as an exclusive residential enclave, however, was not really consolidated until the arrival of James Caulfeild, earl of Charlemont in 1762. Charlemont has been summarized as a 'gentle, cultivated and patriotic nobleman whose chief interests were architecture, scholarship and a version of patriotic whiggery at once gentlemanly and dogged' (Craig, 1948, p. 141). Fresh from an extended grand tour of Europe, he 'resolved on building a handsome city residence, worthy of his classical taste and high position' (*Irish Builder*, 15 February 1894). For that purpose, he chose a site directly opposite the hospital to the north of the gardens which, although John Ensor had prepared a plan for the area as far back as 1755, was still little more than a country track.

It was not until 1769 that it opened as Palace Row while Granby Row, along the west side of the gardens, was opened in 1766. Charlemont employed his friend, Sir William Chambers, whom he had previously engaged to design the Casino at Marino, to execute the plans. Chambers, the author of a noted

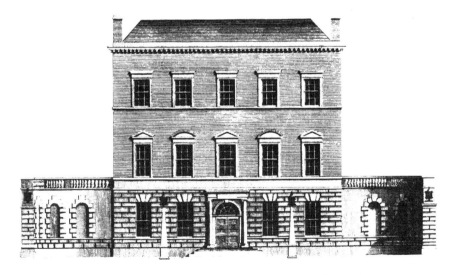

36 Elevation of Charlemont House. (Pool and Cash, 1780.)

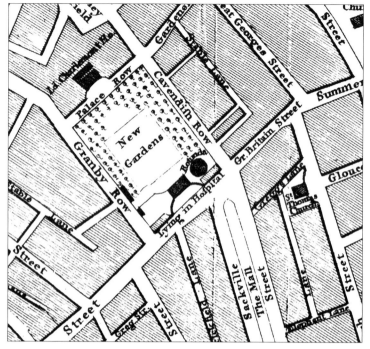

37 Charlemont House and its relationship to the Lying-in Hospital and gardens. (Pool and Cash, 1780.)

eighteenth-century architectural book, *A Treatise on Civil Architecture* (1751), built in what has been described as a modified Palladian style (Summerson, 1986, p. 89). Accordingly, Charlemont House features the characteristic Palladian arrangement of a central villa with two flanking walls sweeping outwards from either side to form a shallow courtyard on to what would become Palace Row (Figures 36 and 37). In a letter to Charlemont, the architect explained the convenience of this arrangement on this particular site, stressing the enhanced relationship of the house to 'the fine prospect' to the south (quoted in the *Irish Builder*, 15 February 1894, p. 15). This 'prospect' was comprised in the foreground primarily by the New Pleasure Gardens and the façade of the hospital. Thus, by the judicious siting of his house, Charlemont was able to enjoy, without any of the associated costs, a relationship between house and garden similar to the one the duke of Leinster had constructed at his property on the eastern periphery of the city.

In fact, Charlemont was also in a position to influence the shape of the Gardens themselves. On 2 November 1759, as a 'Gentleman of Approved Taste' he had been elevated, along with other worthies such as the duke of

Leinster and the Rt Hon. Charles Gardiner, to the hospital's entertainment committee. This had been formed in the wake of Mosse's death to keep abreast of the latest in fashionable entertainment and procure them for performance at the hospital. Charlemont, therefore, could begin to enhance the 'fine prospect' outside his windows. In 1763, for example, Simon Vierpyl – the sculptor Charlemont brought with him from Italy – designed the elaborate new orchestra directly opposite his house on the upper part of the gardens, an intervention which further decorated Charlemont's views while also allowing the lord to enjoy the strains of the gardens' musical entertainments from his own living room. Similarly, it is perhaps no coincidence that the flanking wings which (as discussed in Chapter 1; see Figure 26) complete the garden façade of the hospital building were finally executed around this period, edifying Charlemont's panorama with a Palladian composition as carefully arranged and exquisite as his own.

Since the city of London provided the main source of inspiration for the gardens' entertainments, members of the entertainment committee were presumably chosen in part because of their knowledge of the cultural environment of the capital city. Indeed, it was London which provided the precedent for the gardens' latest and most famous attraction, the one after which the whole hospital complex would ultimately be named. John Ensor's design for the new 'large room', which became known as the Rotunda, was inspired by its namesake in the Ranelagh Gardens in London, which it turn, had drawn from a similarly shaped round building at Vauxhall Gardens. Ranelagh's Rotunda, whose interior and exterior measurements were 150 ft and 185 ft respectively, was reputed by Horace Walpole to have cost £12,000 (Figure 38). In comparison, Ensor's design for Dublin was more modest, measuring only 80 ft in diameter and 40 ft in height and costing £6,044 14*s*. 11*d*., £3,880 of which was paid for by parliament. Unlike Ranelagh, however, the ceiling at Dublin's Rotunda did not have to rely on a central support. Instead, its expanse was held only by the outer walls leaving a completely uninterrupted interior floor space. Part of the Rotunda's *raison d'être* had, like its British cousin, been to lengthen the entertainment season of the Gardens by providing an indoor arena for what were essentially the same activities. The French aristocrat de la Tocnaye described the proceedings during his visit to Ireland in 1796–7.

> They have devised in Dublin a rather singular form of entertainment … It is called a Promenade, and the name made me wish to go and see one. The visitors walk in a circular hall called the Rotunda, and while

there is somewhat more freedom than that which obtains at private entertainments, people only mix with, and speak to members of their own circle. After a certain time a bell sounded, and the company hurried through a door just opened, and groups of friends settled round tea-tables.

(Jacques Louis de Bourgeret, Chevalier de la Tocnaye, trans. Stevenson, 1984, pp 25–7)

Like in the gardens, activities were accompanied by music. The building's round form was broken by a square projection on the west side which provided space, below, for an orchestra and above, an organ loft. Echoing its counterpart in London, the Rotunda's exterior wall consisted of a thick hollow space between two thinner skins of masonry. This space was occupied by a series of niches each 12 ft by 9 ft, decorated with the coats of arms of patrons and accessed directly from the main room. This allowed small parties of individuals to gather and linger in a semi-private realm, discrete from the *mêlée* of the main space. In 1780, it was described as 'one of the finest and noblest circular rooms in the British dominions' (Pool and Cash, 1780, p. 65) with the curving wall of the sumptuous interior articulated with a classically inspired arrangement of a continuous pedestal supporting a series of pilasters surmounted by an entablature. This opulence, however, was not extended to

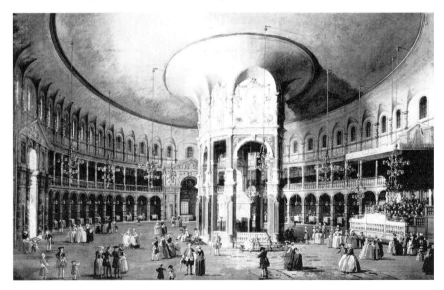

38 Rotunda at Ranelagh, London, interior, mid-eighteenth century. (Antonio Canaletto, 1754.)

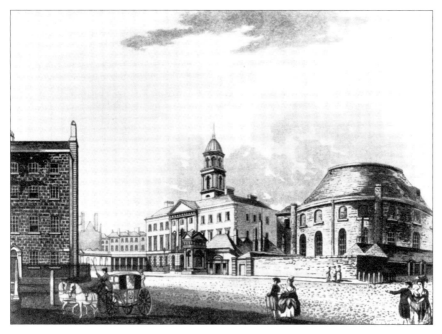

39 View of the Lying-in Hospital and Rotunda (*c*.1770).

the exterior. A print of the Rotunda in 1780 shows a squat, awkward building faced in brick adorned by chimneys and down-pipes and surrounded by an ugly clutter of low structures with pitched roofs (Figure 39). Only later would its introspective nature be altered.

The structure opened with considerable pomp on 5 June 1767 with the event bringing in a return of £173 13*s*., a figure which represented a marked increase on a usual evening's takings for the gardens of about £70. Initially at least, the governor and parliament's speculations about the profitably of additional leisure facilities appeared to be financially justifiable.

What is not clear, however, is precisely what benefits the palatial new hospital and its associated facilities held for the patients. Initially, as the volume of deliveries increased dramatically, so did death rates. The hospital's records allow comparisons. At George's Lane for the entire period of its existence (1745–57), the hospital delivered 3975 women with maternal and infant death rates at 1.1% and 10% respectively. After the removal to Great Britain Street: from the period 1760 to 1766, 3,800 women were delivered with maternal and infant deaths rates of 1.28% and 23% respectively, while from 1767 to 1773, these rates stood at 1.37% and 23.95% respectively. Only after 1774 did the maternal rate fall. The infant rate, however, still remained higher than at George's Lane, a trend which may have indicated a policy towards prioritizing mothers' lives (Kirkpatrick and Jellet, 1914, p. 115). Thus, from 1774 to 1780, a total of 5,903 women were delivered with rates of 1.06% maternal mortality and 19.8% infant mortality. Both rates decreased from 1781 to 1786, when as many as 7,088 women were admitted, with rates of 0.76% maternal mortality and 13.4% infant mortality. These, however, still remained significantly higher than those recorded at George's Lane. Indeed, while comparisons cannot be made with the statistically invisible births taking place outside the institution in houses all over the city, what is certain is that giving birth in the hospital carried considerable risks.

Utility and ornament

In Dublin in 1768, a few months after the Rotunda opened, Edward Foster, MD, an Irish physician trained in Edinburgh, published a treatise in response to an act of parliament which had proposed the establishment of county hospitals throughout Ireland (Act 5. Geo III, c.20, 1765). Foster's *An Essay on Hospitals* praised the general thinking behind the scheme but expressed grave reservations about the form these hospitals were to take which he considered to be borne out of the 'ignorance or prejudice of those instructed to conduct this national charity' (Foster, 1768, pp i-ii).

Instead, the author stressed that all new hospitals should be constructed under scientific principles with their location, construction and administration all being executed according to strict medical and functional criteria. These dealt mainly with the qualities and problems of air and its circulation which, he suggested, could be divided into positive aspects, namely 'purity' and 'dryness' and more negative aspects like 'impurity', 'moisture' and extremes of 'heat' and 'cold'. Accordingly, Foster provided precise guidelines describing where to site hospitals to take full advantage of the former while minimizing the effects of the latter. These included choosing 'a slanting ground of moderate height [with] light, dry, gravely soil [and located] far from mountains, valleys and plains, large rivers and lakes, marshes and ferns, flooded lands, woods, seas and oceans [as well as being] at a distance from towns, smelting houses, lime kilns, manufactories wrought by fire, mines and corrupted, stagnating waters'. He was equally rigorous in pursuing a functional foundation for the prototypical design he included in the text. Significantly, he implied there was a mismatch between the aesthetic concerns of 'architecture' and his own, utilitarian approach.

I have not laid down this Plan to show my Taste in Architecture but to Illustrate my Doctrine by a familiar Example, any little Impropriety in that ancient Science will not be esteemed an Objection to the Propriety of the Design; let not therefore the Execution be rashly censured, until the Intention is impartially considered.

(Foster, 1768, 'An Explanation of the Plates')

The functional requirements of ventilation concerning site and aspect, however, presupposed a distinctly non-urban type of building. The process of appropriating low key domestic premises, the genesis of most Dublin hospitals, was, therefore, summarily rejected by Foster. Instead, standing in isolation within the landscape, yet sheltered by topography and judicious plantings with an adjacent garden for the patients to walk in, his new type of hospital was, externally at least, deeply reminiscent of the country villa and demesne (Figure 40). Unlike the big house, however, internal spatial differentiation was primarily based on medical needs rather than social protocol. For example (as discussed in Chapter 1), Leinster House and indeed the Lying-in Hospital, both contained large, elaborate staircases which connected the public rooms of the ground floor to the *piano nobile* above, whose use would tend to be limited to their aristocratic residents, ceremonial occasions or visiting grandees. Both these buildings contained other, smaller staircases which were discrete and unadorned, connected all floors and tended to be used primarily by serving staff. In Foster's scheme, however, there were two principal staircases, each as wide and as visible as the other which were located at either end of the building and served all floors (Figures 41 and 42, compare with Figures 25 and 27).

A similar concern for medical criteria is evinced elsewhere in the plan. All domestic facilities, such as kitchens and laundries were placed on the ground floor because Foster considered that area to be the most damp and least airy. The first floor – which in a villa would be the important *piano nobile* – was dominated by wards with one large and four small ones, as well as the 'Manager's Room', the 'Apothecary's Appartment' and perhaps most intriguingly, an 'Appartment for the Electrical Machine' (Figure 42). On the second floor, there was an 'Operation Room' with a skylight, and a 'Room for the Dead to lie in'. Opposite, one end of the other wing was to be kept empty, so it could, 'if a contagious Disease should happen to break in the Hospital, be ready to receive either the Clean or the Infected, as either might be least numerous'. Foster specified that no hospital should be more than three storeys high as it was believed that noxious 'Vapours and Exhalations' tended to grow

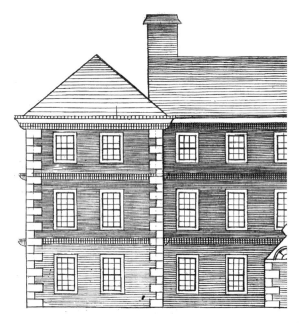

40 Elevation of Foster's 'utilitarian' hospital (detail). (Foster, 1768.)

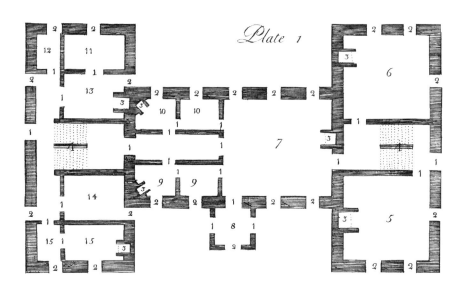

41 Ground Floor Plan of Foster's 'utilitarian' hospital: **1** Doors, **2** Windows **3** Fireplaces, **4** Stairs, **5** Kitchen **6** Apothecary's Shop **7** Admission Hall **8** Porch **9** Porter's Apartments **10** Directress's Apartments, **11** Cold Bath **12** Necessary House **13** Wash Room **15** Steward's Apartment and Office. N.B. Foster does not state what No. 14 is. (Foster, 1768.)

THE HOSPITAL AND THE SPECTACULAR CITY

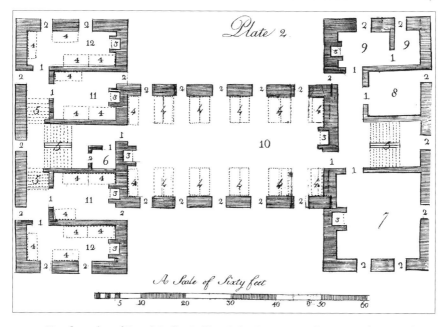

42 First floor plan of Foster's 'utilitarian' hospital: **1** Doors **2** Windows **3** Fireplaces **4** Beds **5** Stairs **6** A Closet for Urinals Etc. **7** Manager's Room **8** Apartment for Electrical Machine **9** Apothecary's Apartments **10** Large Ward, containing 20 Beds **11** Two small Wards containing three Beds each **12** Two small Wards which may contain 2, 3, or 4 Beds each. (Foster, 1768.)

more concentrated as they ascended. Moreover, the larger wards in Foster's design enjoyed cross-ventilation, an arrangement he suggested should be attempted wherever possible.

> [Hospitals should be] single Houses, with numerous Windows on each side opposite to each other; by which means a Renovation of fresh Air is in our Power … were the Houses double, from the necessary Partitions running along their Middles … this Circulation could not be procured.
> (Foster, 1768, pp 26–7)

Ventilation also necessitated a simplicity of design. The author eschewed, for example, the 'over-large wings' which render the '[S]tructure more complicated and prevent the Access of free Air'. Perhaps most significantly, however, was the subject of ornamentation which incurred his special wrath. Not only could it prevent free air flow, but the expense of providing a profusion of elaborate ornament he insisted, 'sink[s] the whole charity into a mere "vox and praeterea ni-hil" – I may say, a deceitful, empty sound'. This critique of magnificence was further emphasized later in the text when he suggested that 'charity is mere ostentation unless proper attention is paid to the applicant of the sums destined to the Purposes of Public Utility' (Foster, 1768, p. 40).

An Essay on Hospitals has been described as a 'new way of writing about hospitals in the English-speaking world' (Stevenson, 2000, p. 125). Foster's suggestion that hospitals could do much more than merely contain, but rather, their location and architectural form, when combined with effective administration and hygienic discipline could actively cure, represents the beginnings of the final stage in Foucault's process of medicalization (Foucault, 2000). Here, empirical scientific method has extended its remit from body to building to become the generator of design. Architectural form and space are accordingly relegated to assume subordinate roles as mere conduits of function, carefully disposed to channel the principal medical requirements of ventilation and medically prescribed spatial segregation. Foster even suggested hospital chapels be disenchanted to take on a more utilitarian role, doubling-up as operating rooms and vice-versa. Such an injection of reason should perhaps have signalled the beginning of the final shedding of *ancien régime* associations and non-scientific practices. Despite these aspirations, however, Foster's pursuit of an architecture of utility, failed to break completely with aesthetic prejudices and traditional conventions. The H-plan form of his design while portending the apparently scientifically predicated shape of future institutions, was still heavily indebted to the Palladian villa. Wrapped in the architectural envelope of a big house, his functionalist hospital appears to apply a scientific post-rationalization to a tradition of building already well established. Indeed, the solid, immutable qualities of architecture may have actually had a considerable influence on notionally scientific medical thinking. It has been suggested, for example, that the eighteenth-century obsession with ventilation was related to the fact that it could be effected by architectural means in a way that other means of avoiding disease 'such as scrubbing and chemical prophylaxis did not' (Stevenson, 2000, p. 160).

If Foster's blend of scientific rationalism, expounded by a solitary physician in the rarefied environment of a treatise, was still infused with traditional aesthetic prejudices, then what of a real-life hospital where these inadequacies were augmented with a whole series of other eighteenth-century social pressures? Although we can see hints of its application in Dublin and elsewhere throughout the second half of the eighteenth century, the position of special scientific knowledge in hospital design was not universally consolidated in Great Britain and Ireland until after the mid-nineteenth century when Florence Nightingale effectively revolutionised the theory of hospital construction by publishing her seminal text *Notes on Hospitals* (Stevenson, 2000, pp 234–5 and Taylor, 1991, p. 8). Until then, aesthetic, political and economic motives had at least as much of an impact on the form of hospitals as medicine. These more partisan concerns, however, were often given a pseudo-scientific or functional veneer. A discussion, for example, took place throughout the eighteenth century concerning the seemingly paradoxical concept of the utility of ornament. Indeed, it was to this very theory that the Revd Lawson appealed, when justifying the magnificence of the Lying-in Hospital. Needless to say, the chapel where he made his speech never witnessed the spilling of guts and blood from a surgical operation.

> [W]hy such grandeur? To relieve these poor objects 'tis right, but why in a palace? You will agree that such building should be large enough for convenience, strong for lasting, neat and warm for health. Now, allow fully for these conditions; ornament occasions a much less additional expense than is imagined; neither is it useless; it gives pleasure to a beneficent mind to behold the seat of the bounty clean, fresh, even elegant; it draws attention and inquiry to a scheme so reasonable and benefitious. Virtue should be beautiful as well as beneficial.
>
> (Lawson, 1759)

Elsewhere in the Lying-in Hospital, however, other schemes which did not have the same visual impact as the chapel were being shelved due to apparent lack of funds. An out-patients department was set up in 1771 after being proposed by Mosse's nephew Thomas, the hospital's chaplain. It occupied the former apartment of the chaplain to the east of the main hall and was soon augmented by an apothecary's dispensary. On 5 April 1777, however, the board decreed that it be closed, 'on account of the Expense of it to the charity'. It is difficult to understand how expensive this scheme would have been as all medical and surgical officers received no wages, medicines were not generally expensive and it was set up in a space already owned by the hospital. It did, however, subvert the established hierarchy of the building by placing poor women in the very areas which hitherto they had been discouraged from entering. Other cutbacks to the hospital's care for patients are also recorded. In the 1780s, for example, due to an increase in the number of patients seeking admission, Mosse's original directive that 'Every Woman is to have a warm decent Bed to herself' was contradicted. The board admitted in 1785, that for some months sixteen beds had been doubly occupied. In addition, the length of stay for recuperation and recovery had been cut from fourteen to seven days (*Journals of the Irish House of Commons*, 7 February, 1785).

Mortality rates in the Lying-in Hospital remained high until Joseph Clarke, (assistant master 1783–6 and master 1786–93) introduced ideas concerning ventilation and a stricter hygienic discipline. Hitherto, not only had windows been sealed, but women had been confined to four-poster-type beds surrounded by heavy fabric to eliminate any possible movement of air in their vicinity. Furthermore, the wards had been constantly heated. Borrowing ideas on ventilation from Charles White's *Treatise on the Management of Pregnant and Lying-in Women* (1773) Clarke carried out very simple measures such as the opening of windows, the boring of holes in the doors and creating openings in the ceilings of each ward in an attempt to increase the movement of air. This appears to be the first instance of empirical medical theory being applied to the built fabric of the Lying-in Hospital. And when John Howard, the eminent prison reformer, visited as part of his tour of lazarettos, hospitals and prisons in 1788, he was impressed. Ventilation had been further increased by the removal of the 'testers' (the fabric walls of the four poster beds) and Howard described the institution as being 'quiet and clean', the 'furniture new' and 'the greatest attention paid to the patients' (Howard, 1791, p. 83). These measures, however, proved futile when dealing with the deadly puerperal (or childbirth) fever. In 1787–8, there was a particularly severe outbreak which, it seems, can be traced paradoxically to Clarke's own spirit of scientific enquiry. As chief demonstrator in anatomy at Trinity College and, like all eighteenth-century doctors, largely ignorant of antiseptic precautions, it has been suggested that Clarke introduced the infection to the hospital himself, when attending births immediately after performing a dissection (Campbell-Ross in idem, ed., 1986, p. 153). Nevertheless, the cheap and low-key interventions by both Clarke and the Revd Mosse appear to have represented some tangible betterment of patients' conditions. As non-spectacular improvements, however, they bore testimony to the impotency or even danger of magnificence in the realm of medical care. Within the political and ideological arena, however, the 'ceremonious but inept architecture' (Foucault, 1991, p. 278) of the hospital continued to be an effective and potent vehicle.

Colonizing the landscape of care: other hospitals in mid-eighteenth-century Dublin

The purpose-built hospitals of mid-eighteenth-century Dublin tended to, in their façades at least, closely echo the architecture of the Palladian villas of their aristocratic sponsors. In this they differed from their counterparts on the British mainland which often only superficially resembled Palladian mansions and retained significant differences. The London Hospital (1753), for example, while displaying the characteristic Palladian features of an emphasized centre-piece and two similarly treated side pavilions, dispensed with the interior arrangement of the villa where different floors represented different degrees of social importance (Forty in King, ed., 1980, p. 70; Figure 43). Instead, the *piano nobile* is conspicuously missing and the building consists of three storeys containing similar functions simply stacked on top of each other. The plan, moreover, shows signs of being predicated according to the way in which the hospital was to function rather than aesthetic demands. Thus, working or medical spaces such as the 'apothecary's shop' and the 'bleeding room' were located just off the main hall occupying conspicuous and public positions within the building's layout.

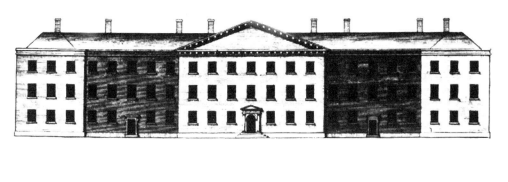

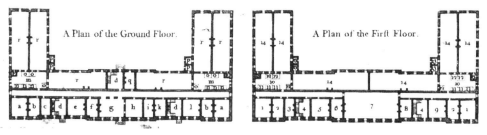

43 Plans and elevation of the London Hospital. (Boulton Mainwaring, 1752.)

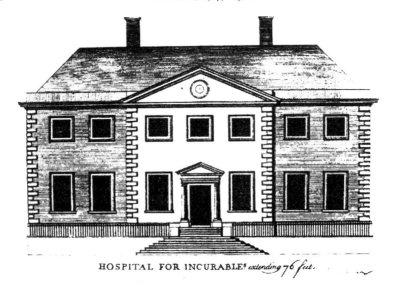

HOSPITAL FOR INCURABLES *extending 76 feet.*

44 Elevation of the Hospital for Incurables. (Engraving after J. Aheron, 1762.)

Such an explicit relationship between a form and spatial organisation influenced by medical practice did not emerge in any meaningful way in Dublin until towards the end of the eighteenth century. Instead, mid-century hospitals such as St Patrick's (established in 1743) and the Incurables (opened in 1754 in Lazar's Hill, Figure 44) retained close approximations of the Palladian villa both in their front elevations and, in the latter example, its interior layout which shows only slight evidence of being influenced by functional requirements.

However, St Patrick's Hospital, a lunatic asylum supposedly influenced by the infamous Bethlem Asylum (Bedlam) in Southwark, London, was more of a hybrid. It has been suggested that the figure of the madman was at the vanguard of the techniques of surveillance and spatial segregation which later characterised most carceral, clinical or reformatory institutions (Foucault, 1993 and Stevenson, 2000). At St Patrick's, the architect, George Semple echoed Bedlam's layout by arranging cells side by side in rows, accessed by distributing galleries. This facilitated supervision and the division of the inmate population into small groups or even single individuals. It was not, however, necessarily predicated on medical or reformatory grounds. At Bedlam, for example, the incurables' wing had an identical layout to the area reserved for those considered redeemable. Compared to Bedlam, St Patrick's arrangement of two wings perpendicular to the front range was even more constraining and

THE HOSPITAL AND THE SPECTACULAR CITY 91

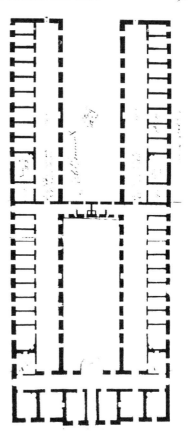

45 Ground floor plan of St Patrick's Hospital, shown here with an extension of extra cells by Thomas Cooley, 1778. The U-shaped plan allowed such extensions to the rear while allowing a close approximation of a Palladian villa in its front façade. (Thomas Cooley, 1778.)

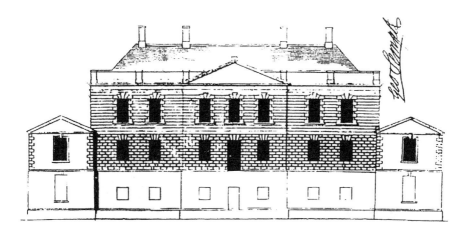

46 Elevation of St Patrick's Hospital. (George Semple, 1749.)

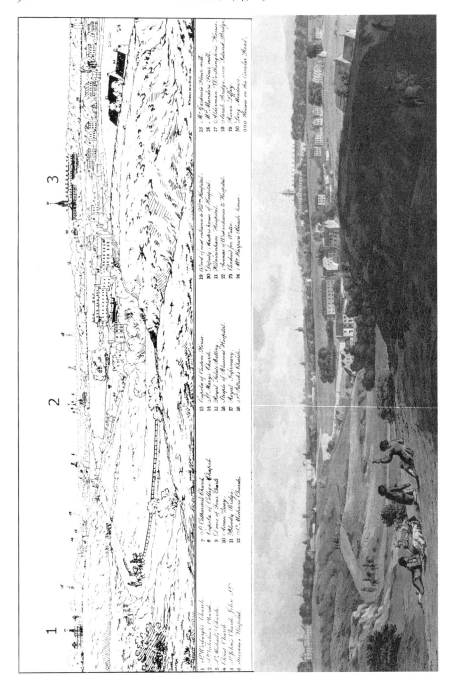

47 Schematic of Malton's view of the city from the west: **1** Royal Military Infirmary **2** Steeven's Hospital **3** Royal Hospital, Kilmainham. (James Malton, 1797.)

patients' freedom of vision was extremely limited: views from the windows of the gallery were purely of the windows of the gallery opposite (Figure 45). However, this arrangement meant that from the public street (Bow Lane), the building read like a Palladian country villa. Moreover, when compared to the vast public frontage of Bedlam, St Patrick's front façade was relatively small in area, a quality which allowed a significant economy by limiting the requirement for expensive cut stone (Figure 46).

The nearby Steeven's Hospital, however, was not built in a Palladian idiom at all, but rather followed a resolutely old-fashioned style which has been described as 'the last kick of the seventeenth century' (Craig, 1992, p. 97). Designed by Thomas Burgh and opening in 1733, Steeven's anachronistic architecture can partly be explained by its proximity to the Royal Hospital, Kilmainham in the city's westward reaches. Superficially at least, its arrangement around a courtyard, its spire and its location seem to play a hierarchical game of form with its larger and more elaborate sibling on top of the hill. It is a relationship which effectively places Steeven's building within a colonial landscape. Designed by William Robinson, the Royal Hospital was built in the 1680s on what has been described as 'a historically conspicuous and topographically prominent site' to the west of Dublin (Olley, 1992, p. 65). The hospital's massive scale and location made it clearly visible from certain key points in the city and its surroundings; from Kilmainham village, from Thomas Street on the route out of the city and, perhaps most importantly, from the main road westwards and the former vice-regal lodge (which subsequently became the Magazine Fort) in the Phoenix Park. In a painting by Thomas Bate in 1685, the Royal Hospital is viewed from this last location as 'a figure in the landscape, a monument set against the horizon spread with the towers and spires of the burgeoning capital' (Olley, 1992, pp 65–66). And, by the time James Malton painted his *View of Dublin* from the Magazine, Phoenix Park in 1795, the Royal Hospital had been joined on the horizon by the Royal Military Infirmary, built in 1788. Together, these two sentinels frame the view of the city with Steeven's Hospital in the middle of the painting further emphasizing the domination of the western approaches to the city by institutions ostensibly dedicated to care (Figure 47).

However, the figures of soldiers galloping on horseback in the middle ground of Malton's print, when combined with the buildings' grand scale and prominent locations, reassert a colonial presence and remind the viewer that the landscape is simultaneously one of power. In fact, the domination of this physical landscape was reinforced by the simultaneous appropriation of an historical one. The Royal Hospital was constructed close to the site of the Priory of the Knights Hospitallers, a medieval, militant religious order given to works of charity for the sick and decrepit. These associations gave the hospital additional potency as a political icon: it recast a site traditionally associated with Catholic care as one of Protestant munificence. Indeed, this quality was not lost on the founders of some of Dublin's eighteenth-century voluntary hospitals. Of Dublin's three medieval hospitals, St John's (1188), St Stephen's (1230) and St James's (*c.*1220), the last two provided the sites for Mercer's Hospital and the Hospital for Incurables respectively.

This kind of appropriation had, as a necessary correlative, the production of history, the reshaping of the past. As the century progressed, a new interest in ancient Ireland developed, reaching a peak in 1785 with the foundation of the Royal Irish Academy. In 1786, Mervyn Archdall, member of the Royal Irish Academy and chaplain to the Rt Hon. Francis Pierpoint, Lord Coyningham, published his impressively titled, *Monasticum Hibernicum, or a History of the Abbeys, Priories, and other religious houses in Ireland; interspersed with Memoirs of their several Founders and Benefactors, and of their Abbots and other superiors, to the time of their final suppression.* Any pretensions the work had to being an objective and academic treatise, however, are somewhat undermined by the author's introduction.

> When we contemplate the universality of that religious zeal, which drew thousands from the elegance and comforts of society to sequestered solitude and austere maceration; when we behold the greatest and wisest of mankind the dupes of a fatal delusion, and even the miser expending his store to partake in the felicity of mortified ascetics: again when we find the tide of enthusiasm subsided, and sober reason recovered from her delirium, and endeavouring as it were, to demolish every last vestige of her former frenzy, we have a concise sketch of the history of Monasticism, and no common instance of that mental weakness and versatility, which stamp the character of frailty in the human species.
> (Archdall, 1786, p. ix)

As the 'deluded' landscape of Catholic care was remade as one of Protestant benevolence, elsewhere in Dublin other, even more partisan political motives were also benefiting from the cloak of legitimacy that the production of history, architecture and visual representation could provide.

The Knights of St Patrick and the Assembly Rooms

The origins of the Assembly Rooms, the last buildings to be added to the Rotunda complex in the eighteenth century, are closely linked to the emergence of a new chivalric order in Ireland, the Illustrious Order of St Patrick. Created in 1782, under the aegis of George III by the Lord Lieutenant George Nugent-Temple-Grenville (second Earl Temple), it has been suggested that the order's inception was essentially political, devised by the British government as part of a strategy designed to curb the power and influence of the Volunteers (Cullen, 1997, p. 67). The latter was a mainly Protestant militia which had been originally set up in the 1770s to defend Ireland – much depleted of its regular army by the American Wars – against foreign attack. By the early 1780s, the British administration was beginning to view the presence of such a large, irregular army of questionable loyalties as a threat to its sovereignty on the island. Consequently, the executive in Dublin Castle set about dismantling the movement, partly by deepening and consolidating its internal divisions and partly by providing a counterpoint to the Volunteers' military displays and parades in honour of William of Orange – perhaps best exemplified by Francis Wheatley's painting 'A View of College Green with a Meeting of the Volunteers on 4 November 1779 to commemorate the Birthday of King William' (1779–80) – which periodically took place in the streets of Dublin and other towns and cities on the island.

Instead, in what has been described as an act of cultural re-orientation, the British established a new focus of ritual and spectacle in the figure of St Patrick, a pre-reformation saint who appealed to both the Protestant and Catholic tradition in Ireland (Cullen, 1997, p. 67). The aristocratic leaders of the Volunteers, Lord Charlemont and the second duke of Leinster (the first having died in November 1773), were among the first to be offered membership in the Illustrious Order of St Patrick. Most significantly, however, was the fact that the highest position, that of grand master, was reserved for the lord lieutenant, the figurehead of British rule in Ireland. The subordinate role that the leaders of the Volunteers accepted in the upper echelons of the order were echoed in the first public spectacle to mark its creation, the inaugural St Patrick's Day parade, which took place on 17 March 1783. Here, the rump of the Volunteers were present but played only a minor role, lining 'the streets through which the procession passed' and keeping order at the service in St Patrick's Cathedral (*Dublin Gazette*, March 1783). The event, moreover, infused with religious and historic meaning, created a potent public image whose significance had the potential to reach beyond any mere military show of force.

> [T]he magnificence of the ceremony, the crowds of spectators of the first distinction in the cathedral and the myriads of all ranks of people in the streets to see the Knights, etc., pass and repass in their carriages to and from the castle, with the animation that lit up the countenances of the public, formed a scene that is indescribable, and which will long be remembered with pride and satisfaction by thousands of the sons and daughters of Hibernia.
>
> (*Dublin Evening Post*, March 1783)

The subsequent celebrations took place in two discrete venues: on 17 March in the ballroom (which Temple renamed after St Patrick) of Dublin Castle, the ancient seat of British rule in Ireland, in the old part of the city, and, on 18 March, at the Rotunda, a site not only closely associated with Charlemont, Leinster and the Volunteer movement, but also at the heart of Dublin's new northern suburb. The scale and import of the event was not lost on the Lying-in Hospital's patients. They were evicted from their wards and attended at home for a few days as the entire hospital complex was requisitioned for the Knights, their retinue and associated entertainments. The hospital received £300 for the event (the usual fee for the Rotunda being £50) and was temporarily re-converted very neatly and easily into a house of hospitality ('Accounts Abstract for the Hospital, 1784', Rotunda Hospital Records).

Over the next three years, the Volunteer force was gradually disarmed by regular government troops. The illustrious Order of St Patrick, however, was to be given a permanent presence in the city. On 4 April 1784, a series of drawings for a new set of rooms, marked with the order's motto (*Quis Seperabit, 1783*) and emblem, were presented to the Lying-in Hospital's board of governors. The author of these drawings was Frederick Trench, resident of No. 2 Palace Row, member of parliament for Queen's County, governor of the Lying-in Hospital, amateur-architect and recently elected Wide Streets Commissioner. On 8 June 1784, after a donation of £400 by the incumbent lord lieutenant, the duke of Rutland and his wife had brought the available funds up to £1,000, the decision to go ahead with the scheme was taken. Accordingly, on 17 July 1784, the foundation stone for the 'New Rooms' was laid by Rutland on the plot of ground immediately to the east of the Rotunda and a building committee consisting of Leinster, Charlemont, Luke Gardiner, David La

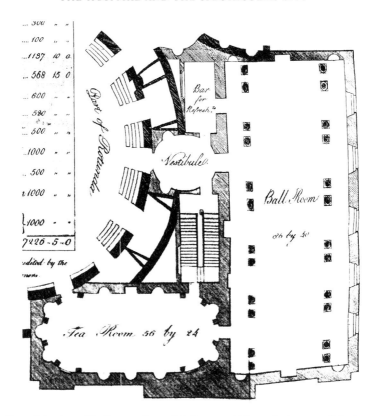

48 Plan of the Assembly Rooms. Cavendish Row would be at the bottom of the image. (Richard Johnston, c.1785.)

Touche, William Bury, Frederick Trench and Dr Rock was established to oversee construction ('Hospital Minutes', 17 July 1784, Rotunda Hospital Records).

The drawings of the New Rooms were sent to the prominent architect James Gandon for comments. Soon after, but not before the foundation stone had been laid, Trench relinquished his position as architect to Richard Johnston. Johnston, however, retained the essence of Trench's design. On appointment, his brief was to produce a full account of money spent and received and 'an Estimate for completion and a full set of drawings on which to base an application to Parliament' ('Hospital Minutes', 11 October 1784, Rotunda Hospital Records). A printed drawing, headed 'The Expence of the Designs underneath is estimated at £9,000, the Funds intended to be appropriated for said work amount to £7225 5s. 0d.,' and signed by the new architect, was produced as part of a document entitled 'Rotunda Hospital Report, 1785' (Figure 48). It shows two rectangular two-storey blocks, one

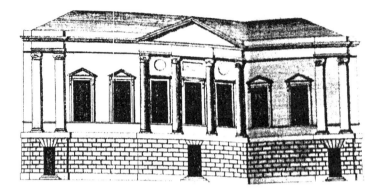

49 The Cavendish Row elevation of the Assembly Rooms. The single unified façade belies the two, differently orientated, spaces behind. (Richard Johnston, *c*.1785.)

larger than the other, arranged perpendicularly and located at the north-east quadrant of the Rotunda. The larger block, running in an east-west direction contained a Supper Room above a grand Ball Room, both measuring 86 ft by 40 ft. It was connected to the Rotunda by a single storey oval vestibule covered by a glass roof.

The smaller block contained another Supper Room measuring 56 ft by 24 ft on the upper level and a Tea Room of the same dimensions below. Both these rooms were connected by a doorway with their counterparts in the larger block. Wedged between the Rotunda and the corner formed by the two blocks, a staircase connected the upper and lower levels. Despite containing two sets of discrete spaces orientated in different directions, the two blocks were united on the public front of Cavendish Row with a single, Palladian style façade (Figure 49).

Not shown on Johnston's drawing was the Card-room built in the space between the Rotunda and the Hospital building. Also omitted, but shown on a set of plans submitted to the earl of Buckingham, lord lieutenant in 1788, was a new entrance to the whole complex, attached to the Rotunda on its southern apex (Figure 50). A description of the interior, revealing the full extent of its connection to the Knights of St Patrick, was published in an account of a masquerade ball given by the 'Gentlemen of Hughes's Club' by Faulkner's *Dublin Journal* in 1787.

> The Ball-room was everything that could be expected. Over one of the chimney pieces was a brilliant girandole composed of the insignia of

the different ornaments of the Knights of St Patrick. This had a splendid and beautiful effect, and the temporary pillars were ornamented with artificial flowers, and festoons of evergreens which hung the whole room and gave it the appearance of simple elegance. The Card-room was fitted up as a refectory, ornamented with festoons and artificial flowers and in the niches were placed orange and rose trees in full bearing. When this room is finished, it will be very beautiful. The vestibule between the Rotunda and Ball-room is covered with a light and elegant canopy of glass, by orange trees, and natural and artificial flowers. The Rotunda was newly beautified, and over the entrance to the Card-room was a transparency of a Knight of St Patrick, at full length, in the habiliments of his order. A complete band in the Orchestra, which was relieved by a regimental one. The supper rooms were more brilliant than could be fully expected from their unfinished state. A few strips of painted paper, were hung up, and were at once an ornament, and imitated the stile in which it was intended to complete the rooms. On this paper were represented a girandole standing on a pedestal, over which was a harp, encircled by a laurel leaf, and over it all a curtain disposed in imitation of a canopy, under which were the initials S.P.Q.H. *Senatus populus que Hiberniae*, the Senate and People of Ireland, in imitation of the S.P.Q.R. of the Romans.

(*Dublin Journal*, March 1787)

For Leinster, Charlemont, Shannon, Mornington, Arran and the lord lieutenant, all governors of the hospital and Knights of St Patrick, the decision to build the rooms was perhaps partly an act of self-flattery which they also extended to the other knights. The earls of Bective, Tyrone, Clanbrassil and Drogheda, for example, all knights of the order but not hospital governors, all contributed financially to the venture (Craig, 1948, p. 195). However, like the decision to build the Rotunda, the Assembly Rooms project was firmly grounded in financial considerations. In 1784, the 'Clear Profits' from the Summer Concerts (£380 1s. 10½d.), Balls in the Rotunda (£63 13s. 4½d.) and the chapel (£81 5s. 11½d.) were markedly lower than the previous year of £581 12s. ½d., £273 16s. 3½d. and £153 16s. 0d. respectively ('Abstract of Yearly Income …', Rotunda Hospital Report, 1785, Rotunda Hospital Records). According to a governors' report, the decrease in income was the result of the inadequacy of its rooms of entertainment. Indeed, as amusements had graduated from one-off events and temporary installations to the Rotunda (which

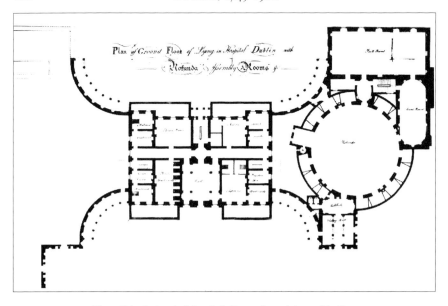

50 Plan of the Lying-in Hospital, Rotunda and Assembly Rooms.
Note the new rectangular entrance at the south of the Rotunda.
(Drawings presented to the earl of Buckinghamshire, 1788.)

had required a much larger and riskier financial speculation), the governors were learning (like future generations of capitalists also would) that investment in the fixed capital of the built environment was particularly subject to devaluation. Physical form and solid masonry were not easily adaptable to the fickle nature of the market place.

The spirit of optimism among the Anglo-Irish following the political concessions of 1782, coupled with the extra wealth generated through the Free Trade agreement, was gradually transforming other parts of the city into areas of glittering spectacle. The novelty and uniqueness of the fifteen year old Rotunda with its dowdy exterior and the considerably older pleasure gardens, was therefore, beginning to fade. Accordingly, the governors proposed the New Rooms keep abreast of the latest fashionable developments, 'to procure … General Intercourse of Society and the Nobility, Gentry and Strangers' ('Appeal to the House of Commons …', undated, Rotunda Hospital Records) and follow 'the Style and Refinement of the present Taste' (*Journal of the Irish House of Commons*, 7 February 1785). The recent huge public interest in the knights of St Patrick and the correlated passion for 'Irishness', made the Order an appropriate theme. Indeed, the article in *Faulkner's Journal* cited above, pointed out that the new rooms were to be completely furnished using only

Irish produce, echoing the lord lieutenant's decision to specify only Irish cloth for all the knights' regalia and gowns. Like the Rotunda, however, the new rooms took developments in England as their precedent. Programmatically, they were very similar to the assembly rooms in York (begun in 1731) which had been designed by the aristocrat and architecture enthusiast, Richard Boyle, third earl of Burlington, the so-called 'father of British Palladianism'. Other links with English precedents were also acknowledged. A publication in 1787, for example, proudly informed the public that the New Assembly Rooms, measuring 19,654 square feet (1,826 square metres) were only twenty feet short of 'the facilities at Bath' ('Sedan Chair List', 1787, Rotunda Hospital Records). It has also been suggested, moreover, that much of Johnston's interior decorative details were taken directly from the latest pattern book designs published by the eminent Scottish architects Robert and James Adam in 1778 (O'Casey in Campbell-Ross, ed., 1986, p. 89).

In fact, the formula for the new rooms was remarkably similar to the one Mosse had adopted decades previously, namely, the enduring appeal of proximity to nobility in a magnificent backdrop of the latest fashionable architecture combined with perennially popular amusements such as eating, music, dancing and playing cards. It was on to this template that the iconography of St Patrick, – already manufactured to channel the potentially dangerous passion for Irish history into more innocuous forms of entertainment and spectacle – was liberally applied. Like other phenomena before it at the Lying-in Hospital, the order of the Knights of St Patrick was recast as an attraction, a fashionable *accoutrement*, a source of potential profit. And like before, this involved a correlative plan of marketing and publicity. Drawings were produced of the architecture and interior design of the new rooms to attract sponsors and raise funds. Some, like those prepared as part of a petition to the marquis of Buckingham showed the Order's iconography *in situ* – in this case, including a miniature portrait of the marquis as a knight. In 1785, a 'List of the Forty Ladies and Sixty Gentlemen, original Subscribers of One Thousand Guineas, toward building additional Rooms to the Rotunda' was published. The presence of many of the esteemed knights, coupled with the attraction of free admissions for Ladies and half-price for Gentlemen to 'six annual charitable *ridottos* … as soon as these Apartments can be completed' helped to induce a whole host of lords, ladies and commoners to subscribe to the rooms. These were supposed to form a fashionable vanguard to attract other potential investors. A note at the end of the list informed the public that the list was to be extended to 150 and that interested parties, 'will be admitted

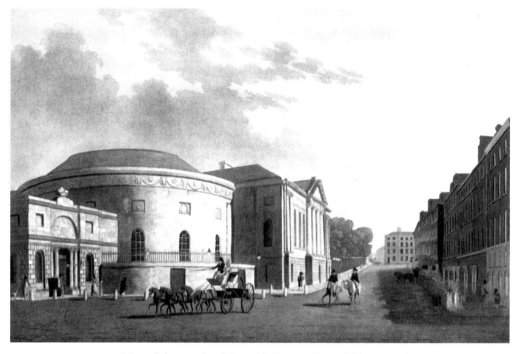

51 View of the completed Assembly Rooms. (James Malton, 1797.)

to the former Terms on Application to the Secretary of the Lying-in Hospital' ('A List of the Forty Ladies and Sixty Gentlemen ...', Rotunda Hospital Report, 1785).

Despite these incentives, however, construction was sporadic and financial problems plagued the scheme from the very beginning. On 22 January 1785, the governors were forced to deny allegations that hospital funds had been used for the new rooms while pregnant women had been refused admittance. On 19 May 1787, building work ceased completely due to lack of funds. A parliamentary grant made more money available, but on 1 May 1789, the entire building committee resigned. It has been suggested that some of the financial difficulties were linked to the decision, taken in 1780, to extend the power of admittance to Roman Catholic clergy. This measure resulted in a rapid increase in the number of admission and the resultant overcrowding fuelled the rapid spread of a puerperal fever epidemic in 1787. Moreover, the decision to evacuate the patients to the coffee room in Granby Row effectively curtailed the gardens' revenue for the season – a loss compounded by the destruction and costly replacement of 'infected' furniture (O'Casey in Campbell-Ross, ed., 1986, p. 82). On 29 February 1788, Trench presented a

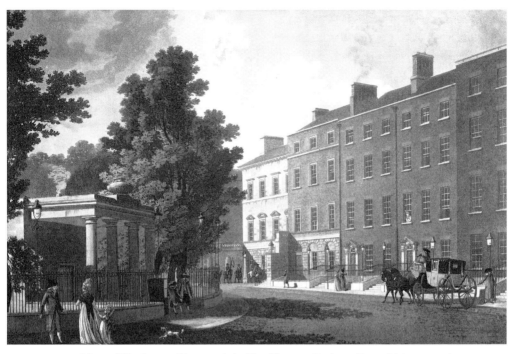

52 View of Charlemont House and the New Pleasure Gardens. (James Malton, 1797.)

report to parliament, stating that £1,116 5s. 11d. was owed to workmen for completed works on the Assembly Rooms. Total expenditure was at this point £11,180 10s. 9d. The final cost of the building would be £15,558 9s. In 1790, parliament allowed the governors to issue £11,000 worth of debentures which allowed works to continue. And finally, on 24 December 1791, the committee reported that the rooms were 'in a state nearly complete' (Figure 51).

The emergence of Rutland Square

Meanwhile, some of the earlier fund-raising methods were having unexpected and far reaching consequences. An act of parliament passed in 1784, for 'the more effectually Paving, Cleansing, and Lighting of the Streets of the City of Dublin', resulted in the taking down of the wall surrounding the gardens and its replacement with a dwarf wall and railing. This was paid for by the square's residents by a tax of 1s. 8d. per foot per annum on the frontage of their houses. Charlemont, whose house frontage was 100 ft (30.5m) and had, in comparison to the other plot sizes of either about 30ft (9.1m) or 50ft (15.2m), by far the greatest tax. Failure to pay resulted in the retention of a section of the wall immediately opposite the offenders' house until they were shamed into acquiescence. 8*d*. of the 1*s*. 8*d*. per foot levy went directly to the hospital and the rest was used to pay for lamps and paving around what had been renamed Rutland Square.

Residents now not only had a closer visual relationship with the gardens, they also had a financial interest in the management and control of the public space immediately outside their houses. The measures, however, did not provide enough revenue to pay for the new rooms and, on 29 April 1785, Trench presented a 'Bill for the completing and effectually lighting and watching of Rutland Square, and for the better Support and Maintenance of the Hospital for the Relief of poor Lying-in Women' to the House of Commons. It became an act of parliament ('Trench's Act'), after amendments, on 19 July 1785. It has been suggested that the bill represented the culmination of Mosse's previous attempts to have the hospital recognized as a national institution. Henceforth, it was to receive an annual income of more than £300 from a tax raised on private sedan chairs in Dublin, collected by the governors of the Foundling Hospital and passed on after deductions. The act allowed the hospital to mortgage the license and raise funds not exceeding £5,000 towards the completion of the new rooms. It also allowed the realization of one of Mosse's other dreams. Grand Juries of all Irish counties were giving permission to raise, in alphabetical rotation, £30 sterling to support the training of a midwife at the hospital (Campbell-Ross in idem, ed., 1986, p. 48).

Malton's painting of Charlemont House in 1793, taken from the viewpoint of Cavendish Street, visualises all the implications of the 1784 and 1785 acts (Figure 52). The pleasure gardens are surrounded by railings articulated every few metres by lamps which also stride rhythmically around the outer edge of the square in front of the houses. Here and there figures stroll on the paved surface. In the foreground an elderly man leans on a cane in front of the garden wall and converses with a woman and child. Behind them, two men are chatting by a sedan chair. Taking into account Malton's propensity for producing slightly sanitized visions of urban life, the idyllic nature of the scene shown here, was perhaps also conditional on the small pavilion with stark Doric columns shown straddling the boundary of the gardens and the street. This was the watch-house established to permit permanent surveillance of the square and gardens. It has been surmised that the 'watching of Rutland Square' proved burdensome to the governors and, therefore, the Police Act of 1786, which absolved their responsibility by establishing a more centralised system of 'watches', would have been welcomed (Campbell-Ross in idem, ed.,

1986, p. 48). However, a petition to parliament from the 'Inhabitants and Proprietors of Rutland Square' in response to the above Bill, suggests it was not the governors who took responsibility for managing the square, but the residents themselves. Moreover, it seems this duty was not unwelcome.

> [We] have, under Statutes now in Force, an absolute and exclusive Right to the Management and Regulation of their Watch, distinct from the City or County of Dublin, or any Parish or other Division; and have effectually maintained a Constable and Eight Watchmen, who are [equipped] with Fire-Arms … at an annual Expense of ONE HUNDRED AND TWENTY-EIGHT POUNDS.
> (Rotunda Hospital Report, 1787)

Paradoxically, the taxation measures introduced to support the hospital helped to create an identity for the neighbourhood distinct from the institution. The financial stake the residents had in the taking down of the pleasure gardens' wall and its replacement with railings, when combined with the unifying effects of the new lamps and paving on the surrounding streets as well as the renaming of the area as Rutland Square, seemed to forge a proprietorial ethos which was at once exclusive and autonomous. Indeed, the square had a larger number of grandees than any other in the city. Of the 200-odd individuals who paid the sedan chair tax specified in Trench's 1785 act, 31 lived in Rutland Square, as compared to 24 in St Stephen's Green and 14 in Merrion Square (Craig, 1992, p. 142). Within this grand assembly, however, only two hospital governors, Charlemont and James Alexander, remained resident in the square. Surrounding properties, long since let or sold by the hospital, were now outside its direct control. Indeed, this manifested itself in a marked lack of enthusiasm for the New Assembly Rooms. Of the total of 48 residents listed in 1785, only seven (including Charlemont and Alexander), were listed as contributors.

Perhaps inspired by the parliamentary autonomy of 1782, the residents of Rutland Square wished to retain a control of their immediate environment which was independent not only from the hospital, but also from the rest of the city. In this last respect, they failed. A document dated 28 March 1786, described the outcome of the residents' petition to retain the authority to police their own square stating that, '[I]t was judged extremely inconvenient to have a District exempt from the regular Jurisdiction of the Police' ('March the 28th', *Rotunda Hospital Report*, 1785). Interestingly, the document also stated that only some of the residents signed the petition implying a difference of opinion among the square's inhabitants. One reason for this schism is suggested by a subsequent paragraph which described some of the financial implications of retaining the square's autonomy.

> The Assessment now payable, is at the Rate of One Shilling per Foot, running Measure, which will cease at the 29th September, 1786; when an Assessment, at the Rate of One Shilling and Sixpence in the Pound of Minister's Money, will take place under the Police Bill. To the tenements of the most considerable Extent in Front, the Police Assessment will be less than at present: To the Generality of the Houses, it will be an Advance of Sixpence per Foot running Measure. So very inconsiderable a Difference of Annual Expence could be no Object. The Protection of the Garden-Railing, and the Indemnity from Injuries, occasioned by the Negligence of the Watch, were the Motives for such Application.
> ('March the 28th', Rotunda Hospital Report, 1785)

Thus, it was in the financial interests of the likes of Charlemont, who had the most 'considerable extent in Front', to have the control of the square devolved to a central authority. Charlemont's personal interests aside, however, that such a distinguished lobby group as the residents of Rutland Square should be denied in their petition perhaps testified to the influence of another, more powerful group operating in Dublin, one whose authority would ultimately reshape the city's entire eastern half.

The Wide Streets Commissioners

In 1769, John Bush had suggested that if Sackville Street was extended to the river, it would become 'one of the grandest and most beautiful streets perhaps in Europe' (Bush, 1769, p. 11). By the mid-1790s, not only had this happened but Rutland Square and Sackville Mall had become part of a series of magnificent spaces which swept across the River Liffey to College Green and from there to Dublin Castle. These developments were the result of the effort of an extra-governmental body called the Wide Streets Commissioners (hereafter WSC). Originally established in 1757, 'to make a wide and convenient Way, Street, or Passage from Essex Bridge to the Castle of Dublin', the WSC's influence was subsequently extended until, by the end of the century, they had dramatically transformed the appearance of central and eastern Dublin.

The extension of Sackville Street began in the 1780s. Central to the plan was the relocation, first mooted in 1774, of the Custom House further downstream to the east of Sackville Mall. The political implications of this will be discussed in more detail below, but for the moment it suffices to know that the move happened and the foundation stone of the new Custom House was laid on 8 August 1781. Similarly, the decision to build Carlisle Bridge was resolved in 1782 as was the decision to continue the line of Sackville Street northwards to break into Dorset Street and create North Frederick Street. In addition, on 16 December 1785, it was resolved to extend Sackville Street to the Liffey and, in 1790, it was decided 'to carry Westmoreland Street in one line from Carlisle Bridge to the House of Lords' (McParland, March 1972, p. 18). D'Olier Street was created about the same time, fanning out south-eastwards from Carlisle Bridge towards the other end of Trinity College, creating a wedge of building between itself and Westmoreland Street. These developments effectively made Sackville Street the principal north-south axis of the city, providing a wider and more ceremonious alternative to Capel Street (Figure 55; see Sheridan in Brady and Simms, eds, 2001, pp 108–35).

The art-historian Edward McParland (1972, pp 1–32) draws our attention to the apparently organic and shambolic city shown in *Rocque's Plan* of 1757 and contrasts it with the series of ordered and uniform façades characteristic of the WSC's interventions. The process by which the new streets were made involved the compulsory purchase of properties, their subsequent demolition and the dissolving of previous patterns of boundary and ownership. The streets were then widened to a minimum width of not less than 100 ft, followed by the construction of buildings with façades stretching over the new boundaries, seamlessly linking discrete dwellings and properties. Dame Street,

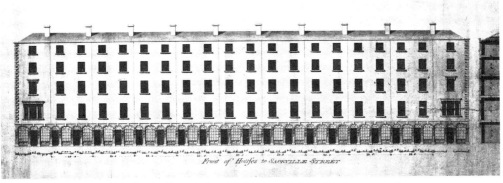

53 Wide Streets Commissioners' elevations in Sackville Street extension. (Thomas Sherrard, 1789.)

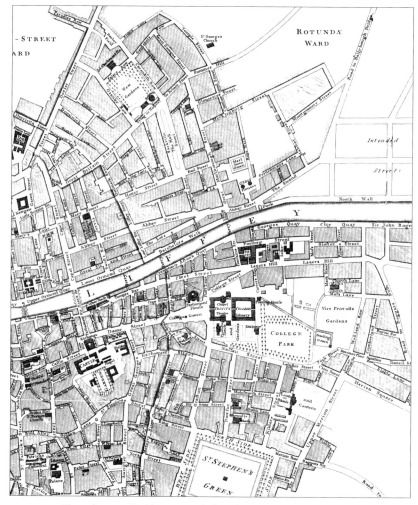

54 Plan of eastern Dublin in 1780 before the extension of Sackville Street to the river. (Pool and Cash, 1780.)

Westmoreland Street, D'Olier Street etc., all displayed these characteristics, as did Sackville Street's extension to the river (Figure 53). However, on *Rocque's Plan*, Sackville Mall, with its orthogonal geometric form, copious length and width, was already conspicuous in a landscape of irregular and narrow streets. Therefore, while the WSC extended the street, no widening was necessary. Similarly, the regularity of the new extension merely complemented an existing regularity in materials, scale and openings in the older part of the street. Moreover, the WSC's techniques of purchase, demolition and reconstruction, echoed the way Luke Gardiner had made the Mall in the first place, decades earlier.

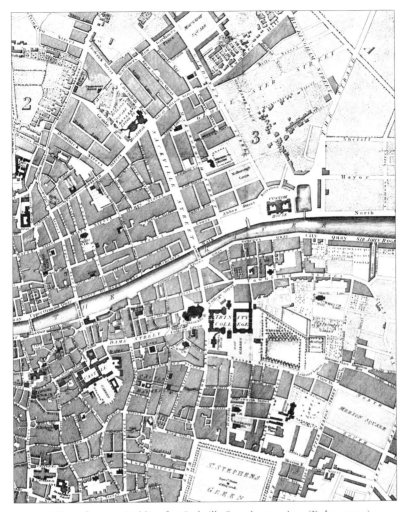

55 Plan of eastern Dublin after Sackville Street's extension. (Faden, 1797.)

It would seem, therefore, that Sackville Mall provided a key influence on the way the city was remodelled under the WSC and perhaps even formed the template for other planned developments such as Merrion Square and the Fitzwilliam estate in the 1760s (Walsh in Dickson, 1987, p. 36). McParland (1972, p. 9) also suggests that Sackville Mall's earlier alignment with College Green was not merely fortuitous, but rather, 'the eventual Westmorland Street scheme of the WSC may have had its origins in the plans of the first Luke Gardiner', thus representing an earlier, aborted attempt to realign the city eastward. Perhaps fittingly, Gardiner's grandson, also called Luke, was one of the commissioners who ensured its ultimate realization. By the end of the century, Sackville Street had become merely one constituent part of a network of wide and regular streets which formed the new eastern city, embodying the transformation of a section of Dublin, from Arthur Young's (1780, p. 6) description of the 'narrowness and populousness of the principal thoroughfares' into what has been termed an 'idiosyncratically grand city' (Foster, 1988, p. 188).

As shown in Chapter 1, mid-century Sackville Mall resembled a theatrical space. Its width and straight lines allowed the gaze to wander and its broad surface became the stage on which the leisure classes could participate in daily performances of spectacle and display. In this, it was following a historical model. It has been suggested that, beginning in the fifteenth century, the conceptual boundaries between urban and theatrical space became blurred. In response to a chaotic urban environment inhabited from medieval times, Renaissance humanists such as Alberti began to propose that the highly ordered world of the theatre was an appropriate model for urban design. He conceived of an ideal city as an imaginary theatre of 'tragic scenery' where the streets were paved and perfectly clean and lined with two identical rows of houses or arcades and porticoes of uniform height. In this 'harmonious work of art' everything would be arranged according to what Alberti considered to be universal laws of order, number and proportion (Boyer, 1996, p. 78). The 'tragic scene', one of a triad of theatrical motifs which emerged in antique theatre (the others being the comic and the satyric), was described by the ancient Roman writer Vitruvius as being characterized by an architecture of nobility: 'columns, pediments, statues and other royal surroundings'. In this scene actions of great importance were enacted because such things, as was later emphasised by the Renaissance architect and writer Serlio in 1545, 'always happen in the houses of great Lords, Dukes, Princes and Kings'.

Under the Wide Streets Commissioners, throughout central and eastern Dublin key civic buildings were either created or remodelled to articulate the new urban spaces with the characteristics of gravitas and the timelessness and permanence of classical architecture. Within the uniform landscape of brick terraces, buildings which interrupted the pattern in materials, plot size and building line, achieved a conspicuous presence. For example, the Royal Exchange built in 1769 of Portland stone by Thomas Cooley and equipped with temple front and portico provided an emphatic termination to the new vista opened up by parliament Street. In 1782, the House of Lords recommended that its own chamber be extended. When Cooley's initial plans were passed over, James Gandon accepted the commission. The significance of his Portland stone Corinthian portico standing proud from the main bulk of the

House of Lords was not entirely realised until the completion of Westmoreland Street allowed it to be viewed against the backdrop of Trinity College and College Green from Carlisle Bridge.

Meanwhile, at the other end of Sackville Street, the dowdy exterior of the Rotunda was undergoing a similar transformation to participate in the new streetscape. The location of the New Assembly Rooms at the narrowing point of the city's new main thoroughfare afforded a distinct visibility which was enhanced by the framing of its mountain granite exterior in a perspective composed entirely of brick. Indeed, Trench's submission of the designs for the New Assembly Rooms in 1784 had actually coincided with his election to the Wide Streets Commissioners, a relationship which perhaps serves to underscore the close connections between such signature buildings, their sponsors and the emerging urban landscape. Three other governors of the Lying-in Hospital, Luke Gardiner, David La Touche and John Foster were also Wide Streets Commissioners and, in an appeal to parliament for more funds for the Assembly Rooms, the hospital governors consciously placed the new project in a wider urban context by emphasizing its potential for 'ornamenting the Metropolis' ('Appeal to Parliament from the Hospital Governors', undated, RHR). Thus, the new entrance pavilion to the Rotunda was oriented to be seen from and engage with Sackville Street. Similarly, the Assembly Rooms gave a coherent classical façade to what had become North Frederick Street (formerly Cavendish Street), the main route north. What was left uncovered of the Rotunda, was also given a more acceptable public face. A 'Parapet and Freeze' was raised around its perimeter and decorated with classical details like bucarnia (ox-head skulls) and swags.

It has been suggested that the WSC's projects were symptomatic of a wider social climate and were grounded in political and cultural motives. McParland (1972, p. 5), for example, has described the interventions as 'the obvious material manifestation of the principles of Grattan's parliament'. Indeed, the major works of the building programme did correspond with the administration's brief flowering, accelerating immediately after 1782 and slowing down in the mid to late 1790s. For others, however, the development of eastern Dublin represented an attempt to establish a discrete Protestant city. Central to this argument is the apparent emphasis of the WSC's interventions – beginning in the 1780s and exemplified by the extension of Sackville Street – on linking the various disparate, privately-owned, affluent Protestant suburbs into a centralized urban vision. The new city of spectacle and 'coherent façade', it has been suggested, was built as 'a mirror in which its dominant elite would see their entire culture reflected' (Campbell, 1985, p. 25). Indeed, it was only in the 1780s and 1790s (that is, once the new works were well under way) that the approving term 'Ascendancy' began to be widely used to describe the Anglo-Irish ruling class. Once again, the immutable qualities of the built landscape seemed to offer a psychological crutch as architectural form became a vehicle to express a stability largely absent from their political situation (Foster, 1988, p. 194).

This echoes the interpretation of Alberti's urban theatre cited above, that is, the desire to create an ordered society by constructing the type of ideal and utopian landscape found only in rarefied conditions. This, of course, is a similar set of aspirations and imperatives to those which helped shape the form of the demesne and the big house of the aristocracy. The series of exclusions, isolation and the unswerving adherence to a single vision necessary to the execution of such a project, however, proved impossible in the public realm of the city. As shall be shown, once created, the static architectural set-pieces of grand new public streets and squares were subject to other, more fluid processes. However, even in the act of creation, the Ascendancy city was the product of a hidden power structure which made it more politically ambiguous and complex than many subsequent writers have realised.

Collectivised self-expression requires co-ordination. Consensus between differing groups and localized interests is not easy to maintain. The historian Murray Fraser (1985, pp 102–21) notes that the administration of late eighteenth-century Dublin fell to three powerful but conflicting bodies; the aristocratic parliamentarians, Dublin's merchant class comprising Dublin Corporation, and the British legislative of Dublin Castle. Citing examples where the British legislative intervened on behalf of both the other groups at differing times, he surmises that it was there that the dominant interest and balance of power lay. The notion that the WSC's developments represented a straightforward embodiment of national pride in the city, the expression of an autonomous Anglo-Irish parliamentary elite is, therefore, simplistic. Instead, Fraser suggests that many of the interventions made by the WSC during Grattan's parliament were actually the result of a closer alignment of Irish interests with those of Great Britain. For example, the decision to award the design of the Royal Exchange (one of the WSC's first developments) to the relatively unknown English architect, Thomas Cooley – a man who was 'well-versed in the latest [English] neo-classical fashion' – is perhaps indicative of a process where British tastes and interests prevailed (Fraser, 1985, p. 105). Similarly, Warburton, Whitelaw and Walsh, the celebrated nineteenth-century chroniclers of Dublin, suggested that the Royal Exchange gave the viceroy, symbol of British authority in Ireland, a visible presence hitherto missing in Dublin. Therefore, Parliament Street, so named to celebrate the impact of a group of patriotically minded Irish parliamentarians on the Irish capital, also spectacularly celebrated the converse of Irish autonomy, an omnipresent British legislative (Figure 56).

> [T]he appearance of the Exchange, in the approach from Capel-street is particularly striking; built on nearly the highest ground of the city, called Cork-hill; it is exposed to sight with considerable advantages and terminates the view with an object, at once grand, chearful and elegant. It is perhaps, the most elegant structure of its kind in Europe, and standing on the north-east angle of the Castle, adds considerably to the grandeur of the approach to the residence of the Viceroy.
>
> (Warburton, Whitelaw and Walsh, 1818, p. 520)

A similar situation existed at the New Assembly Rooms, where the political intrigues surrounding the creation of the order of St Patrick had been given an architectural expression in the exterior decoration chosen by Frederick Trench. For the tympanum of the main façade's central pediment, Trench decided on a combination of the duke of Rutland's coat of arms and the star of St Patrick (Figure 57). This not only publicly confirmed the building's intimate connection with the order, it also emphasized the dominant position of the viceroy as its grand master. Whatever the ambiguities of the Royal Exchange and Parliament Street or the subtleties of decoration at the Assembly Rooms, Fraser contends that it was the new Custom House (1781–91), designed by James Gandon, which represented the clearest example of the influence of direct colonial management in the architecture of pre-union Dublin. Funded directly by the British Government, roundly criticized by Henry Grattan and fashioned in a 'thorough-going neo-classicism', it displayed explicitly in its iconography, symbolic representations of the harmony of union between Britain and Ireland, a fact noted by the artist James Malton in his description of some of the building's architectural details in 1799.

> In the Tympan of the Pediment, in *alto relievo*, is represented the friendly union of Britannia and Hibernia, with the good consequences resulting to Ireland; they are placed in the centre, on a Car of Shell, embracing each other.
>
> (Malton, 1799)

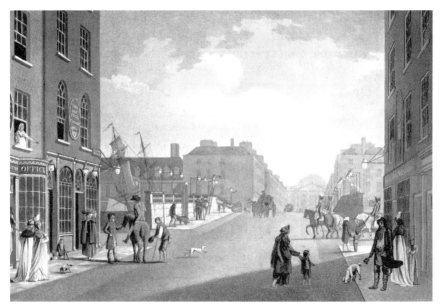

56 View of the Royal Exchange from Capel Street. (James Malton, 1797.)

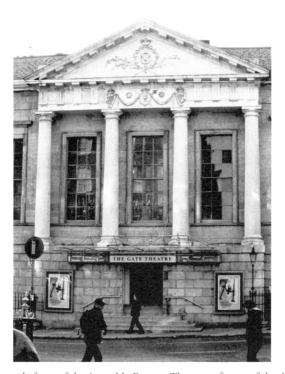

57 View of temple front of the Assembly Rooms. The coat of arms of the duke of Rutland is contained in the tympanum. (Author's photograph, 2002.)

A city divided: the limits of the Wide Streets Commissioners' interventions

It has been suggested that Grattan's 'hyperbole' of patriotic rhetoric often served as a façade to obscure the real nature of things and that the creation of the new city seemed to coincide with a gradual disengagement with political and social realities by the Ascendancy (Foster, 1988, p. 251). Significant as it was, the impact of the Wide Streets Commissioners on Dublin was limited. Almost all of their larger-scale projects in the eighteenth century took place to the east of the old town (Figure 58). Indeed, faced with the problem of Dublin's squalid and decaying medieval fabric, the Commissioners chose to extract what was deemed important from it and effectively ignored the rest. Thus a series of linking moves unfolded to make the Castle more visible and emphasise its symbolic link with the eastern city whose centre was focussed on College Green. After Parliament Street had been opened up in 1762, the route connecting the Castle to College Green and parliament was reinforced. This occurred when an act, passed in 1781, widened Dame Street in order to 'to open a suitable avenue between the seats of the executive and legislative bodies' (21 Geo. III, 1781).

Like the other developments, Dame Street was lined with ordered and continuous façades. Behind this thin mask of buildings, however, the squalor of the old town remained much as it was before. The same was true of Temple Bar, haunt of a series of bawdy houses, low theatres and non-conformist churches. Moreover, as the fashionable city expanded eastwards, it tended to leave behind in its westward reaches, its most obvious characteristics of poverty and contradiction. There, one could find in close proximity, a cluster of carceral, reformative and medical institutions: the Soldiers' Infirmary on Thomas Street, the House of Industry, the Foundling Hospital and the House of Correction on James' Street and further west, St Patrick's Lunatic Asylum on Bow Lane and Steeven's Hospital on Steeven's Lane. Unlike the Lying-in Hospital, other institutions for the poor were less easy to accommodate within upper class areas.

Two buildings, both designed by the same architect and constructed in close proximity to one another but on either side of the western limit to the Wide Streets Commissioners' interventions, provide an apt metaphor for the growing division of the city into discrete spheres of spectacle and invisibility. Thomas Cooley originally arrived in Dublin in 1769 to take part in the competition to design the Royal Exchange, the elaborate end piece of the

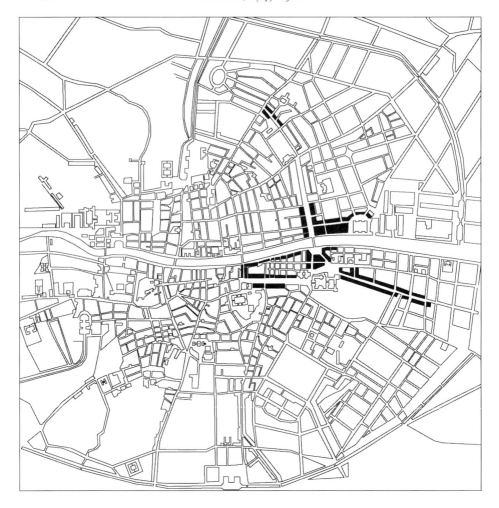

58 The eighteenth-century interventions of the Wide Streets Commissioners. (Compiled by author. Based on Taylor [1816] and Warburton, Whitelaw and Walsh [1818].)

Commissioners' Parliament Street scheme. His winning project became, 'one of the principal ornaments of the city', providing a termination not only to Parliament Street but also, by extension, Capel Street. By virtue of its location, the building's main public façade, a temple front and portico constructed in creamy Portland stone, enjoyed a generous amount of space in front which permitted the play of light upon its walls (Figure 59). However, just beyond the westward side of Capel Street (at what is now St Michan's Park, Green Street), Cooley also designed Newgate Gaol. This building's principal façade,

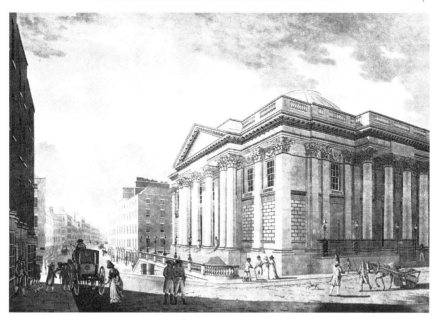

59 Another view of the Royal Exchange. (James Malton, 1797.)

carved in black limestone, abutted other buildings and addressed narrow streets in a cramped neighbourhood of the city untouched by civic improvements (Figure 60). Yet, despite their differences, Cooley's two buildings retained certain similarities in their functions. The Royal Exchange provided one of the scenographic backdrops to the daily theatre of the new magnificent city, whereas Newgate Gaol provided the context for a rather different type of theatricality in the shadowy city beyond the wide streets – the spectacle of discipline and death.

Built between 1773 and 1780, Cooley's Newgate derived at least some of its architectural form from its London namesake which had been designed by George Dance and completed in 1768 (Figure 61). Part of the function of Dance's building was to provide a suitably sombre backdrop for the spectacle of execution in London. It had also been built, however, to replace an older gaol located within the city walls at the New Gate entrance to the city of London. There, felons, criminals and debtors had been held in what Foucault described as 'a prison of the threshold', a 'non-space' between inside and outside the city, a highly visible site where passers-by would be continually reminded of the results of transgression (Foucault, 1993, p. 11). This disciplinary function was transferred into the very façade of the new prison with the constituent elements of terror translated from the display of real bodies into a built proxy, a heavily rusticated exterior wall, embellished with real iron fetters (Figure 62).

Until the last quarter of the eighteenth century, hanging in Dublin had taken place on the so-called 'fatal tree' at St Stephen's Green. The guilty were conveyed there by cart from the old prison, in a centuries-old tradition of 'hanging processions' (Henry, 1994, p. 16). By September 1780, however, this had been replaced by executions at Cooley's new gaol. Similar to London, Dublin's Newgate was built to replace an older 'New Gate' located at the Thomas Street entrance to the city. And, like Dance's design, the 'new'

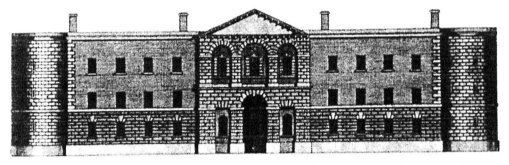

60   Elevation of Newgate Gaol, Dublin. (Published according to an act of parliament, 1779.)

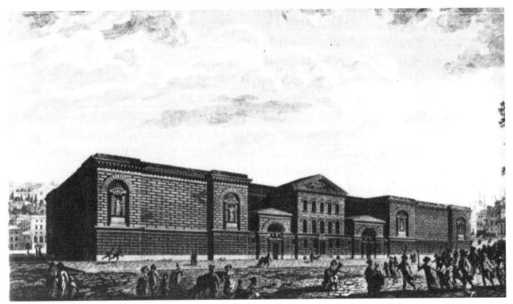

61   View of Newgate Gaol, London, designed by George Dance, 1768. (Ferdinand Bourjet, c.1790.)

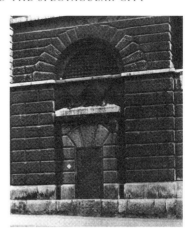

62 Debtor's Door at Newgate, London. (Nineteenth-century photograph in the collection of the National Monuments Record, London.)

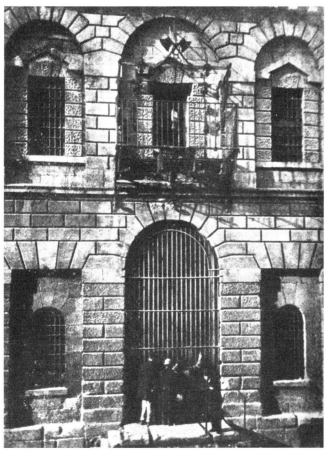

63 Detail of façade at Newgate, Dublin. (Nineteenth-century photograph in the collection of the Dublin Civic Museum.)

Newgate at Little Green, begun in 1773 and completed in 1780, adopted a rusticated façade. By 1783, however, in place of the merely symbolic fetters of Dance's design, Cooley's Newgate was adorned with the actual apparatus of death – the gibbet. The hanging procession was now merely a walk from the cells to the chapel from which the condemned emerged through a window on to the gallows (Figure 63). And while, in the months between executions in London, the scaffolding was removed, in Newgate Dublin, it remained, silently but visibly awaiting a new victim. In both Dance's and Cooley's Newgates, this scenographic function appears to have been the overriding design concern. The spectacle of hanging at Newgate was far more dramatic than anything seen at St Stephen's Green, but it seems that under almost all other criteria, Newgate Jail was considered a complete failure (Henry, 1994, p. 23). In 1782, just one year after the completion of the building, the prisoner reformer John Howard wrote that Newgate represented the 'reverse of every idea … of a perfect and well-regulated jail' (*Journals of the Irish House of Commons*, 1782). Equally, Dance's Newgate in London served to convince Howard 'that prison design would have to be fundamentally rethought' (Markus, 1993, p. 121).

In Dublin, Newgate Gaol was only the first of a series of institutions to arrive on site at Little Green. It was followed by the Sheriff's Prison in 1774, Sessions' House (courtroom) in 1792 and finally, the City Marshalsea in 1804. Located close to the Ormond Fruit and Vegetable market, other places of employment and large amounts of surrounding poor housing, this cluster of buildings provided a disciplinary lesson specifically for the population of a working class area which was discretely hidden from the magnificent urban spaces of the WSC's interventions. Denis Taafe's account of Dublin in 1796, however, reveals that the boundaries between the newly stratified city were more porous than might have been expected. The notion of a 'harmonious city', inspired by the likes of Alberti, where 'everything had its proper place, proportion and order', was completely subverted by spectres of poverty and contradiction.

> The east part of the capital indeed displays some grandeur in palaces, public buildings and works which instead of disguising makes more glaring the huge poverty, the gigantic misery that fills this great city, in every garb, in every shape of human woe and gradation of wretchedness. Every street, every lane every place of public resort is crowded with squalid victims of oppression … pomp and property

alongside abject poverty, such magnificence in building and equipages, coupled with the filth of mud cabins and the rags that disfigure the poor … It is an insult to us in our poverty to withdraw so large a portion of our scanty circulation from more useful channels in order to rival in the pomp of buildings the opulence of London or Amsterdam … your colossal edifices are propped up on our mud cabins.

(Taafe, 1796, p. 14)

Paradoxically, as the seamless façades covered up the neglected zones of the city, the increased visibility in the wide streets made the presence of the poor and destitute all the more conspicuous. However, it was not only the appearance of shadowy figures from 'backstage' Dublin which affected the appearance of the eastern city. Other groups were exiting under pressures of a slightly different kind. A marked decline in the aristocratic profile of Sackville Street's residents in the years following 1790 has been noted. The opening of the street to the river attracted many visitors which made it an ideal location for commerce, a situation which was reinforced by the building of the bridge. This caused the old aristocratic elite to begin to drift to newer, more tranquil areas such as the nearby Mountjoy Square or the Fitzwilliam estate across the river. In turn, their place as residents was taken by members of the merchant and professional classes and their businesses, a process which confirmed the re-orientation of Lower Sackville Street as a predominantly commercial area (Walsh in Dickson, ed., 1987, pp 38–40). Something similar happened in the New Pleasure Gardens, where there was a shift from exclusive court music to entertainments more suited to middle-class tastes in the final two decades before the Act of Union. From 1788 onwards, the declining popularity of the gardens among the upper classes was confirmed. Concerts were reduced to one a week and the last concert organized by the Lying-in Hospital governors was given on 6 May 1791. Thereafter, all concerts were given by lessees (Boydell in Campbell-Ross, ed., 1986, p. 124).

Other, less formal types of commercial entertainment, however, were burgeoning. In 1797, John Magee, proprietor of the *Dublin Evening Post* wrote a scathing attack on the practice of street-walking prostitution in the public streets of the city. He considered the activity to be the 'primary cause of riots, quarrels, nocturnal disturbances, robberies, maimings, and frequently of murders'. His vehemence may have been due to the fact that the problem was 'particularly severe' directly outside his offices at No. 41 College Green (Lyons, 1995, p. xi). It would seem, therefore, that the very heart of the WSC's magnificent and heroic streetscape was subject to the regular occurrence of unseemly behaviour, or, as Magee put it, 'debaucheries, horrible oaths and shocking obscenities'. Magee's solution was not idealistic. Accepting that 'universal chastity in the inhabitants of a capital city is a circumstance rather to be wished than expected', he proposed that a discrete area of the city be set up and dedicated to nefarious activity. Thus 'when evils, from the depravity of the age must, they might be regulated as to do the least possible mischief' (*Dublin Evening Post*, 14 September 1797). In the course of the nineteenth century, an adulterated version of this vision was realised. Dublin did indeed obtain a discrete red light district in the hinterland beyond the main thoroughfares, but, as will be shown, it was informal and unregulated. The exact reasons for its location in the north-east of the city remain unclear. It was, however, in close proximity to one of the most famous and fashionable resorts of sexual licence and louche behaviour of eighteenth-century Dublin: the Lying-in Hospital's pleasure gardens, Rotunda and Assembly Rooms. Similar to the way that public activity and engagement irrevocably altered and compromised the ideal vision of the Wide Streets Commissioners' project, the semi-public realm of the pleasure garden, set in a landscape inherited from the demesne, had provided bountiful opportunities to transgress class, gender and sexual boundaries under the cloak of charity and magnificence.

Dublin and its demi-monde

Sex and the Pleasure Garden

Mrs Delany's description of the 'rude mob' at Mosse's free breakfast in 1751, proved to be one of the milder examples in a string of disturbances and incidents of disorderly conduct at the pleasure gardens which spanned decades. In June 1762, the band of music was 'abused and ill-treated', provoking the governors to order that threats of prosecution be placed in journals and newspapers. This was the first of what was to become a series of attempts to place controls on the behaviour of the gardens' visitors. The following year saw the threats augmented with a reward of twenty guineas for information leading to prosecution and, in 1765, the offer was repeated.

> … it was Resolved that any Person or Persons who shall misbehave by raising any Riot of Disturbance in the Garden, shall be prosecuted at the Expense of the Corporation; and that any Person who shall discover and prosecute such Offender or Offenders, shall, upon Conviction, be entitled to a Reward of Twenty Guineas.
>
> (Faulkner's *Journal*, 1765)

In addition and about the same time, the perimeter wall was raised and topped with broken glass. Meanwhile, in 1764, a handbill addressed to parents was printed compelling them to keep their children under control and prevent them committing 'many Mischiefs by running up and down the Slopes and defacing them, climbing and leaping over the Rails, breaking the Globes and Chairs, running through the Flower Beds, tearing down the flowering Shrubs, and destroying every appearance of Flowers' ('Hospital Minutes', 3 December 1764, Rotunda Hospital Records). Later in the century, parents were asked not to bring children at all. The problems, however, did not go away. In 1785, sixteen years after the directive which forbade the giving of alcohol to patients, a similar order that 'No Malt or Spirituous Liquors, Wine or Cider be sold or supplied to any of the Company in the Rotunda,' was issued. The parliamentary acts of 1784 and 1785, which partly concerned the effectual lighting and paving of Rutland Square were, therefore, also borne out of a very real concern for controlling disorder. The taking down of the boundary wall and its replacement with railings, however, suggests that this concern was in part directed at one specific type of disorderly activity.

In mid-century London, Vauxhall Gardens was already renown as a setting for sexual intrigues. It was a place 'where lovers met in the lamp-lit walks before drifting amorously to the less crowded periphery where mock rockeries and clumps of shrubs covered their flirtations. Here, music from the orchestra floated over them as they kissed and loosened fastenings' (Tillyard, 1995, pp 177–8). Both the plan of 1756 and that of 1764, show a similar densification of planting towards the boundary wall at Dublin's New Pleasure Gardens (Figures 17 and 26 respectively). Moreover, the serpentine walks penetrating the shrubbery offered a variety of secluded corners and discrete dead ends which were isolated from the rest of the assembly. The taking down of the high wall and its replacement with railings and the erection of lamps, as prescribed in the 1784 act, effectively opened these ambiguous zones to closer scrutiny. That this method of surveillance was designed to be executed from outside the gardens, however, is perhaps also significant. It allowed some tightening of control without too much of an aesthetic intrusion. Enough perhaps to curb wilder transgressions while allowing the 'dream-like' atmosphere and more innocuous forms of assignation to continue.

The production of fantasy was crucial to the success of the commercial pleasure garden. However, sexual desire was not only a product of that 'enchanted world'; it was also one of its contributing factors (Ogborn, 1998, pp 116–129). Within a finite space, a heterogeneous assembly, having paid money to experience pleasure, strolled around a landscape where everything was designed as an object of visual attraction. If pleasure gardens offered an opportunity for the upwardly mobile to mingle with the upper classes, then of course, for the aristocracy, the reverse was true. Here, one could mix outside the narrow realm of peers and enjoy especially the company of women of other social backgrounds. As everyday life was temporarily suspended, fuelled by alcohol and music, social and sexual mores were similarly loosened from their restraints.

In 1790, the *Hibernian Magazine* published two illustrations comparing sartorial fashions in 1745 and 1790. Both images show groups of figures, decked in the latest costumes promenading themselves at the city's most fashionable resorts. 'Taste-à-la-mode, 1745' depicts Marlborough Bowling Green and 'Taste-à-la-mode 1790' shows the New Pleasure Gardens. In both illustrations individuals are engaged in the act of looking at one another (Figure 18 and Figure 64).

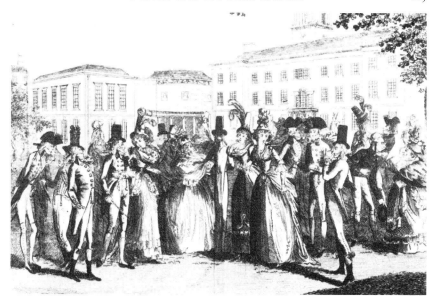

64 Taste-à-la-mode, 1790, the New Pleasure Gardens. (*Hibernian Magazine*, 1790.)

However, in the latter scene, the reduced girth of the hooped skirts and the absence of swords, allow the figures to become more tightly packed together. They have also been given an architectural backdrop, that of the hospital, the Rotunda, Assembly Rooms and the terrace houses on Cavendish Row. These, unlike the trees at Marlborough Bowling Green, confirm an urban quality. Moreover, the buildings' row of windows gazing impassively on to the scene seem to have heightened the potency of the gaze and emboldened the protagonists' behaviour to make their visual *communiqués* more direct and highly charged. A lady engages her foppish companion with a cocked head and frank look. Elsewhere, a man is peering through a monocle at a lady who is evidently not of his company, but is candidly returning his stares.

In London, Vauxhall Gardens had acquired its reputation as a site of sexual adventure as far back as 1712. Other gardens also had a certain notoriety. In 1796, the proprietor of the 'Temple of Flora' lost his license for keeping a 'disorderly house', while 'Lambeth Wells' – a resort which combined 'the pleasures of purging waters and all-night music' – was closed in 1755 due to numerous brawls. Other gardens barely disguised their amorous undertones. Cuper's Gardens, also in Lambeth, for example, was known colloquially as Cupid's (Porter, 1994, pp 173–4). Indeed, this ambiguity was replicated in the generic term for such places: pleasure gardens. In his diatribe on English culture and manners in the early 1740s, Henry Fielding, writing anonymously in the guise of a French visitor, uses the same adjective 'pleasure' in a description of some of England's principal vices: 'Eating, Drinking, Smoking or Making Love to Ladies of Pleasure'. The tract finishes with a withering description of Vauxhall and Ranelagh Gardens and the dubious activities found there (Ogborn, 1998, p. 126).

At the end of the century another, this time authentic, French visitor, de la Tocnaye, published the second edition of his *Promenade d'un Français en Irlande*, which included a more detailed description of some of the activities to be found in the Rotunda, Dublin. Perhaps significantly, the text, which contained the following observation – '… *en un mot je ne doute que cette Promenade ne répondit parfaitement à son objet … d'aider les couches les femmes*' – was not translated into English, (de La Tocnaye, 1801, p. 24). Like the adjacent pleasure gardens, the Rotunda provided a large central area where one could mingle amongst the crowd and observe its attractions while a series of peripheral niches accommodated more discrete liaisons.

The clients and memoirs of Mrs Leeson, madame

The social ether of the pleasure gardens was perhaps at its most potent in the phenomenon of the masked ball or masquerade. By the time the celebrated *Ridotto al Fresco* had reopened Vauxhall Gardens in 1732, such occasions had already been vilified for their immorality and ability to give vent to 'frenetic sexual solicitation' (Ogborn, 1998, p. 128). Under the cloak of disguise, social and sexual freedoms could be pushed to new limits as identities and origins blurred into irrelevance or were revealed or concealed at will. In 1785, at one such masquerade in the Lying-in Hospital's pleasure gardens, the prostitute Peg Plunkett, a.k.a. Mrs Leeson, arrived with 'four of the prettiest *impures* in all Dublin' who she introduced as Venus and the three Graces. For herself she chose the garb of Diana, Goddess of Chastity, explaining that the concept of masquerade required an alteration of character:

> [F]or had I appeared in the character of Cleopatra, Messalina the Ephesian matron or any such, it surely could not be deemed masquerade; as to be in masquerade is undoubtedly to be in an assumed character; thus I sported that of the goddess of Chastity.
>
> (Leeson in Lyons, 1995, p. 147).

Leeson was a *demi-mondaine*, a high-class prostitute who mixed in the upper echelons of Dublin society. She was also the proprietor of a series of elite brothels where guests experienced lavish entertainments, including music, masquerade balls and, at her Wood Street house, 'an elegant garden'. In 1795, after she had been made bankrupt by her former clients' refusal to honour debts, she decided to publish her memoirs. The decision provoked a great deal of anxiety and uneasiness amongst those clients whose louche disposition had hitherto been kept from their families (Lyons, 1995, p. vii). Her intimate knowledge of vice in the city and friendship with other ladies of pleasure ensured that some of those libertines who did not fall into her own personal remit, still found their way into her anecdotes. Amongst her own, personal clientele, however, she numbered a lord lieutenant and a host of aristocracy, merchants and professionals; some of these are already familiar.

Charles Manners, the duke of Rutland, vice-president of the Lying-in Hospital's board of governors, knight of St Patrick and original contributor to the Assembly Rooms (and whose crest still adorns its façade), was described by Leeson simply as 'honest Charley'. She recounted their first assignation at her house in Pitt Street, revealing the audacity of the lord lieutenant in his pursuit of sex as well as his cavalier attitude towards the misuse of government funds.

> [We] were soberly drinking our tea [when] we were surprised with the trampling of horses at the door, and a monstrous tantarara, when behold to our amazement who should be announced but his Grace himself, attended by two of his Aid-de-Camps and a troop of horse, the latter of whom remained on horse back armed cap-a-pee, with swords in hands, from one o'clock in the morning 'till five in the afternoon of the next day, sixteen hours!! to the no small surprise and amusement of the whole neighbourhood, and indeed of the entire city, who all flocked to behold the state, the exalted Peg was worshipped in by the Vice King of the Realm. The Aid-de-Camps soon decamped with an *impure* each, but as for honest Charley, he and I, *tête-à-tête*, drank and spilled three of four flasks of sparkling Champaigne, after which we retired together, for his Grace would take no partner but myself, and in the morning he paid me a profusion of compliments on the happiness he enjoyed in my company … [H]e had me immediately placed on the Pensions List under a borrowed name, for three hundred pounds a year.
> (Leeson in Lyons (1995), p. 144)

David La Touche (III) (1729–1817), Wide Streets Commissioner and governor of the Lying-in Hospital was a regular client at Leeson's Wood Street brothel.

Richard Wellesley (1735–81), earl of Mornington, governor of the Lying-in Hospital, member of its entertainment committee and one of the founders of the Hospital for Incurables, was a client and friend of Mrs Brooks, a prostitute and brothel owner. Thomas Taylour, earl of Bective and knight of St Patrick was a guest at Leeson's (illegal) 'May Day Masquerade' at her brothel in Wood Street, dressed as a drummer-boy while Nathaniel Warren, Lord Mayor of Dublin and Lying-in Hospital governor, was a guest at the same masquerade. Also invited was William Robert Fitzgerald, second duke of Leinster, knight of St Patrick and vice-president of the Lying-in Hospital. He was a reputed lover of Mrs Porter, one of Leeson's former prostitutes, whom she had dismissed for her alleged 'depravity'. Preparations had been at the masquerade for the duke's arrival.

> The supper consisted of every thing the season afforded and money could purchase; it was elegantly laid out in the two-pair of stairs street-room, and with the wines, gave general satisfaction. The back-room, contained the only bed in the house (all the others being removed) and for that bed I had put myself to great expense, the furniture being of a new muslin, richly spangled. It was kept locked up, being designed for the Duke of Leinster, who, after all the preparation, never came.
> (Leeson in Lyons, 1995, p. 94)

Meanwhile, John Fane, earl of Westmoreland (1759–1841), lord lieutenant of Ireland, knight of St Patrick and vice-president of the Lying-in Hospital, was refused patronage by Leeson on account of the cruelty he showed his wife, 'who died of a broken heart in consequence of his connection with that celebrated demy rep the honourable (heaven how that word is prostituted!) Mrs S[innot]' (Leeson in Lyons, p. 151). Other familiar characters mentioned by Leeson include Jan van Nost, who as well being a sculptor, apparently doubled as a private investigator and was hired by one of Leeson's lovers to keep a watch on her fidelity. He found it wanting. Finally amongst the peerage, Lord Bristol, Frederick Augustus Hervey, the bishop of Derry and an adversarial colleague of Charlemont in the Volunteer movement, also puts in an appearance as one of Leeson's personal clients.

For the prostitute, pregnancy and venereal disease were occupational hazards. Perhaps understandably, therefore, Leeson established close contacts with members of the surgical, medical and apothecary professions throughout her career. Charles Bolger was the surgeon at the Lock Hospital, Donnybrook who, according to Leeson, offered the building as a venue for one of her masquerades. She sent for him during her last illness but finding he was in the debtor's prison, had to apply to Mr Brady, an apothecary, for help. Surgeon Vance, despite having no apparent training in obstetrics – he was attending surgeon at the hospital for Incurables in 1771 and at the Meath Hospital in 1781 (Watson's *Almanack*, 1771 and 1781 respectively) – delivered Leeson of a 'a dead-child with one of its legs broke' after an altercation at her brothel. Similarly, James Cleghorn, State Physician and member of the board at the Westmoreland Lock Hospital (Watson's *Almanack*, 1797), was sent for by Leeson after an incident of physical abuse by her lover. On discovering she was pregnant he called in William Collum, the same obstetrician and Master of the Lying-in Hospital (1766–73) who had priggishly argued against teaching at the hospital lest it provoked a 'breach of modesty'. According to Leeson, '[b]y their united care, I at length recovered, with the loss of my child, of which I was above four months gone' (Leeson in Lyons, ed., 1995, p. 49).

Collum's treatment of a known and unmarried prostitute who was perhaps also suffering from venereal disease, suggests that the moral stipulations concerning admission to the Lying-in Hospital were not extended to his own private patients. In fact, midwives in the eighteenth century had a 'long-standing and unsavoury reputation [as] managers of sexual intrigues' or, as one seventeenth-century poet put it, they were 'the truest friend to lechers'. It has been suggested that private and shadowy 'lying-in homes' run by both male and female operatives, like Mother Midnight's house in Daniel Defoe's *Moll Flanders*, existed throughout the century. There, '"ladies of pleasure" or others anxious to keep their pregnancy hidden, might be aborted, or await the birth of their child in secret' (Donnison, 1977, p. 34). In a similar vein, it has also been alleged that the discrete position of the maternity ward in the basement of the Hôtel Dieu in Paris was borne out of a similar desire for secrecy (Thompson and Goldin, 1975, p. 119).

Ambiguities and contradictions at the Lying-in Hospital

At Dublin's Lying-in Hospital, the regulations which publicly announced the necessity of marriage and moral rectitude as a basis for entry are contradicted by the private information contained in the hospital records. Patient registers are often strewn with entries where information including husbands' names has been omitted. These discrepancies tend to accelerate towards the end of the century. For example, out of the first 1,098 entries contained in the patient register book 1791–7 (this figure spanned from the start of the book in May

No.	Woman's Name	Age	Husband's name and business	Parish	Admit.	Deliv.	Observations
1	Judith Rockford	28	John, a labourer	St Andrew	15 March	20 March	Mother and child very well
2	Mary Hughes	33	George, a smith	St Bridget	2 April	20 April	Mother and child very well
3	Cat. McDaniel	25	Randal, a servant	St Andrew	12 April	23 April	Mother and child very well
4	Eliz. Bacon	26	John, a soldier	St Paul	13 May	24 June	Mother and child very well
5	Marg. Clark	30	John, a sawyer	St Andrew	13 May	6 June	Mother and child very well
6	Hannah Schullery	27	Thomas, a pedlar	St Mark	14 May	12 June	Mother and child very well
7	Marg. Kelly	32	Richard, a taylor	St Michael	16 May	10 June	Mother and child very well
8	Bridget Goslin	24	John, a cottoner	St Michael	25 May	3 July	Mother and child very well
9	Rebecca Bagwell	28	Thomas, a weaver	St Paul	29 May	3 July	Mother and child very well
10	Mary Read	20	James, a soldier				Mother and child very
71	Mary Dunsfield	25	Michael, brogue maker	St Audeon	30 Nov	5 Jan 1746	Mother very well. Child dyed 8th day fit.
83	Elinor Grimshaw	26	A drummer abroad	St Andrew	30 Dec	14 Jan	Child dyed soon as born. Mother dyed 5th day of a fever.
97	Mary Keghan		A soldier	St Peter	4 Feb	4 Feb	Still born. Mother went out well.

65 Extracts from the Lying-in Hospital Patient Register, 1745, Rotunda Hospital Records. (Compiled by the author.)

No.	Woman's Name	Age	Husband's name and business	Parish	Rel	Admit.	Deliv.	Observations
30001	Mary Walsh	29	Michael, a servant	St Audeon	RC	4 May	5 May	Mother and child well
30002	Brigit White			St Catherine				
30003	Eliz. Flanagan	27	Thos., a servant	St Mary	RC	5 May	5 May	Mother and child well
30004	Mary Morton	22	Michael, a servant	St Michan	RC	5 May	5 May	Child dead woman well
30005	Marg. Kelly	29	James, a weaver	St Catherine	RC	5 May	5 May	Mother and child well
30006	Anne Byrne	20	John, a clerk	St Catherine	RC	5 May	5 May	Child dead woman well
30007	Eliz. Rourke			St Werberg		5 May	5 May	Mother and child well
30008	Cat. McLoughlin		William	St Werberg		5 May	6 May	
30009	Jane Fitsimons	35	Widow	St Michael Wo	RC	6 May	6 May	Mother and child well
30010	Anne Mathews	23	John, a servant	St Peter	RC	6 May	6 May	Mother and child well
30027	Anne Collin/Bryan			St Patrick	RC	11 May	11 May	Still born woman dead
30077	Cat. Lord			St John		22 May	22 May	Still born
30081	Eliz. Morrison					22 May	23 May	Still born
30136	France Carney	30	Chris, a labourer	St Michan	RC	10 June	11 June	Still born, woman dead

66 Extracts from the Lying-in Hospital Patient Register, 1791, Rotunda Hospital Records. (Compiled by the author.)

until the end of 1791), husbands' names are omitted 89 times (see Figure 66). In 76 of these 89 times the 'Observations' are also missing. In comparison, of the first 1,098 entries contained in the first register (1745–56) at the old Lying-in Hospital at George's Lane, only 22 examples fail to give the husband's name and even then always give his occupation. Similarly, there are only six omissions in the 'Observations' column (Figure 65).

More intriguingly is the fact that of the 13 entries which gave 'Observations' but no husbands' names in the 1791–7 register, almost every one represented a fatality: 13 child deaths and seven women's deaths (with two entries stating that the women and child were well and two entries that the women 'ran away') out of an overall general total of 101 child deaths and 17 women's deaths. The general mortality rates for the sample are 9.2% for children and 1.5% for women. Out of this, 11.5% of the children's death rates and 41% of maternal death rates are from entries where no husbands were given. In comparison, in the sample from 1745 to 1756, there were 83 child deaths and ten women's deaths giving rates of 7.6% and 0.9% respectively. Where no husband's names where given, there were only four child deaths and two maternal deaths, giving rates of 4.8% and 20% respectively. In both samples, therefore, entries with missing information have far higher maternal death rates and in the 1791–7 sample, this discrepancy is extended to the infant death rates.

There are a number of possible explanations for these anomalies. Firstly, information about the patient may have been gathered in the period after the birth. Therefore, deaths during labour would have prevented the registrar from obtaining the relevant details. This, however, is contradicted by both the convoluted admissions procedure (described in chapter 1 above) and the few remaining admission forms found in the hospital records. Ostensibly these forms were required to be presented to gain entry. Along the bottom of each, the husband's name, occupation and religion have been clearly hand-written (Figure 67). Moreover, there are entries in the samples where despite the woman dying, full information was still recorded, see for example, Entry No. 30136 in Figure 65. However, there may have been humanitarian reasons for some of the discrepancies. The discovery of a pregnant woman in the city, for example, too ill to undergo the usual admission's procedure, may have induced the hospital authorities to waive convention. Her subsequent death in their care would leave a series of blanks in the records.

The increase in omitted information in the 1791–7 register can also perhaps be contributed to the massive increase in the hospital's turnover of patients. The sample 1,098 in 1791 spanned from May to December. In the 1745–6 register, the same number of patients took until 1749 to pass through the books. Nevertheless, the comparison between the two registers reveals a marked decline in the recording and accumulation of information, which has been regarded as one of the cornerstones of scientific method (Foucault, 1977, pp 189–91). Indeed, this lack of development in the hospital records runs contrary to the accepted trajectory where medical science tended to steadily and progressively exert its presence on hospital management towards the end of the eighteenth century and especially after 1790. Therefore, Wilde's

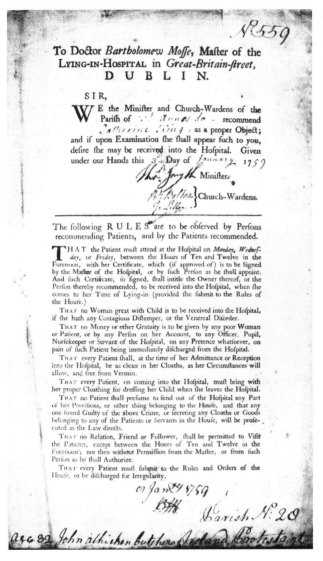

67 Lying-in admission certificate. The age, name, occupation, country of origin and religion of the patient's husband is handwritten along the bottom of the page. (RHR)

observation that the register of 1745–6 was ahead of its time no longer applies to the register of 1791–7. Like other phenomena at the hospital, this shift can possibly be attributed to the transferral of control after Mosse's death, from a professional surgeon and obstetrician, into the hands of a board of governors and guardians which contained only a minor medical or surgical representation. The burgeoning city, however, also contributed to the diminishing statistical visibility of the patients. Entries giving a husband's name, profession and address as 'John, a labourer, [the parish of] St Patrick' may have sufficed in the

Dublin of 1745. But by 1791, the vast increases in population meant such entries no longer had the same precision. Instead, on discharge, patients and their new charges could vanish into relative obscurity in densely populated and more anonymous parishes.

Confusion in the hospital registers also meant, however, that any abuses in the admissions process could be more easily concealed. In fact, the opportunity to by-pass set procedure had been there almost since the beginning. In an undated mid-century letter from Mosse to 'the Lord Mayor, Sheriffs, Commons, Citizens of the City of Dublin', petitioning for funds and support, Mosse reminded his correspondents of one of the benefits of being a guardian, governor or benefactor: the power of admission.

> [R]egard shall always be paid to Certificates or Recommendations of poor women from the Lord Mayor or Recorders of this City, or from any one of the aldermen or sheriffs, or any two of the common council.
> (RHR)

The discrepancies in the records may suggest abuses of the hospital admissions procedure but they do not necessarily indicate that those prostitutes or women of louche disposition who frequented the gardens outside were also accommodated as patients in the hospital or, indeed, made up the anonymous or incomplete entries in the hospital register. The gentry who associated with prostitutes tended to do so mainly with those in the upper echelons of the profession (Lyons, 1995, p. ix). High-class courtesans like Leeson tended to receive handsome recompense for their services and, as we have seen, could afford private medical treatment. But the marital infidelities of the gentry were not always restricted to ladies of pleasure. In 1751 Emily, wife of James, the first duke of Leinster, and pregnant by him for the fourth time in four years, wrote to her sister describing how her husband's extra-marital activities had led to the simultaneous pregnancy of one of their household servants.

> I must tell you by the way of n.b. that things can breed in this house as well as her Lady K[ildare]. You will hear more soon – and 'tis to be hoped that my turn for getting a lover will come in good time.
> (quoted in Tillyard, 1995, pp 99–100)

The aristocratic household, like the pleasure garden, accommodated a cross-section of social classes, concentrated within the confines of a single dwelling. Such an environment of proximity, imbued with a hierarchical and patriarchal power, was a fertile site for seduction and the abuse of authority. In comparison to 1745–56 register, the 1791–7 register shows a marked increase in the proportion of husbands' occupations listed as servants which, it has been suggested, would imply their spouses were also in service (Brophy in Dickson, ed., 1987, p. 53). Governors may have used their powers to ensure their own servants or servants of friends received preferential admission. Such distortions, however, could easily be extended to ensure the results of any of their own moral transgressions be discretely dealt with. Mosse's scheme to provide foster homes for children born at the hospital would have ensured the results of such hiccups could be quietly disposed of forever, without resorting to the horrors of the Foundling Hospital.

Tension and desire in the Lying-in Hospital chapel

The Lying-in Hospital chapel was a space of ambiguity. The interface between the benefactors and the patients, it hints at hidden complexities in their relationship and invites a series of interpretations. Like often happened in the chapels of 'big houses', it simultaneously produced a relationship of proximity and separation, ordering its congregation into two discrete zones based on class, and in this case, gender (Revd Lawson's addressing the congregation as 'Christians, Citizens and Men' suggests its majority was male). It was a space of veneration which focussed on the fecundity of women and motherhood. High above the congregation, the patients' galleries were placed within the context of a highly ornate ceiling containing images of pure moral virtue. Moreover, as can be seen in the drawings made for the marquis of Buckingham in 1788 (Figure 27), the lower pews were arranged perpendicularly to the altar so that, instead of forming part of the congregation's peripheral vision, the upper galleries assumed a visual prominence. Like the Theatre Royal, the gaze of the spectators was not necessarily concentrated on the stage or altar.

As discussed earlier in chapter 1, as well as being a space of worship, the Lying-in Hospital chapel was also a special feature in the New Pleasure Gardens – that fantastic landscape which was characterized by objects of visual delight and where the gaze was often loaded with sexual desire. Unlike the candid stares of the gardens, however, visual interaction in the chapel was more circumspect. In the dimly lit space, the gauze of the balconies' twisted wrought-iron railings obscured the movements of the swollen figures above and disguised individual identities. While encouraging a visual and aural connection between the predominantly male congregation below and the female patients above, the architecture of the chapel simultaneously underlined the division between them. Within the atmosphere of sexual availability of the pleasure gardens, to experience such an abrupt expression of physical separation while enjoying visual and aural intimacy may have contributed to an atmosphere of teasing, sexual tension. However, the sexual profiles of some of the hospital governors, combined with the irregularities contained in the hospital registers, hint that the prohibitions stressed by this space had, at other times and places, already been transgressed.

It is tempting to suggest these ambiguities are also implied within the chapel's decoration and iconography. In *De Architectura*, Vitruvius assigned human personalities to the architectural orders (Figure 68). The Doric exemplified 'the proportion, strength and grace of a man's body', the Ionic was characterised by 'feminine slenderness' and the Corinthian imitated 'the slight figure of a girl'. This personification altered slightly during the Renaissance. While Scamozzi echoed Vitruvius in his description of the Corinthian as 'virginal', Sir Henry Wotton, writing in 1624, labelled the order, 'lascivious' and 'decked like a wanton courtezan'. More than a century later, John Aheron's *A General Treatise of Architecture in Five Books*, the first book to be printed on architecture in Ireland and published in Dublin in 1757 (the year the Lying-in Hospital moved to Great Britain Street), provided a similar interpretation.

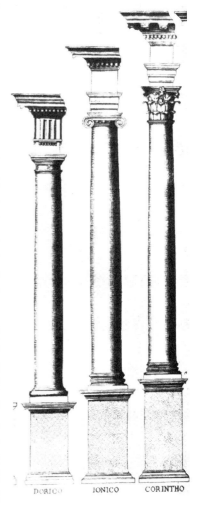

68 The three orders, from left to right: Doric, Ionic, Corinthian. (Serlio, 1611.)

> The Doric Order is the Gravest and preserves, in comparison with those that follow, a more masculine Aspect. The Ionic Order represents a Kind of feminine slenderness, not unlike a light Housewife, but in a

decent matron-like Dress. The Corinthian is a column lascarously decked like a Courtezan, and therein participating (as inventions do) of the Palace where they were born. Corinth having been without Dispute, one of the wantonest and luxurious Towns in the World.

(Aheron, 1757, pp 56–7)

All three orders are represented in the Lying-in Hospital. The temple front dominating the main southern façade is formed by the Doric, as is the portico on the garden side and the columns and entablature in the main entrance hall. The Ionic forms the Venetian windows on both the north and south façades as well as articulating the tower. The Corinthian, however, is reserved for only one place in the hospital: the chapel. Here, Corinthian columns support the women's gallery (Figure 69), and the Ionic columns, which form the Venetian window on the exterior of the south façade, are replaced on its inside by Corinthian ones.

While the limited, internal use of the Corinthian perhaps reflected issues of cost and durability, the order's elaborate capitals make an appropriate addition to a space covered by a dense layer of iconography. The baroque style, which at first seems so out of step with the hospital's austere Palladian exterior, is curiously

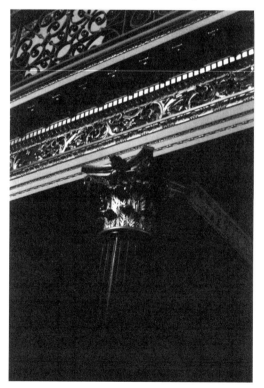

69 View of Corinthian column in the Lying-in Hospital chapel. (Author's photograph.)

appropriate to a space at the intersection of a complex patterning of so many, often contradictory, meanings; space of worship, veneration, proselytising, spectacle and desire. This simultaneity precludes a single, unequivocal interpretation. The chapel's effusive decoration accordingly creates a dream-like atmosphere which oscillates between fantasy and reality while belonging entirely to neither: a space of imagination, interpretation and appropriation.

The Magdalen Asylum and the Bethseda chapel

The Lying-in Hospital chapel, however, was not the only institutional space to position an upper class congregation in close proximity to a group of working class female 'inmates'. The chapels in the Magdalen Asylum in Leeson Street, established in 1766 by Lady Arabella Denny (grand-daughter of William Petty, author of the *Down Survey*) and the Lock Penitentiary (Bethesda), established in 1794 by William Smyth and the Revd John Walker, both created a similar relationship. The focus here, however, was not on 'the tender Mother and the faithful Wife,' but rather:

> [Those] unfortunate females abandoned by their seducers and rejected by their friends, who were willing to prefer a life of penitence and virtue to one of guilt, infamy, and prostitution.
> (Warburton, Whitelaw and Walsh, 1818, p. 771)

Visitors to the Magdalen chapel were admitted by ticket only and, 'since it was the only place of worship in the vicinity, it was patronized by some of Dublin's elite' (Peter, 1907, p. 18). Initially the penitents were barred from the services, but by 1770, a new and larger chapel had been built, allowing them to participate but only as an unseen presence. The incumbent Dean Bayley described the arrangements in his sermon at its opening on 18 March 1770.

> [the chapel was enlarged] so that the worship of God might be celebrated with propriety and order, that a reasonable number might be contained in it, and that the penitents might have a convenient place to join in the service of God, and receive the instruction that may be offered to them without having any communication with the rest of the congregation, either in their entering or retiring from the chapel.

The Dean's oratory continued – in what is perhaps a thinly veiled attack on the Lying-in Hospital chapel – to criticize the misuse of architectural ornament and decoration. Instead, he celebrated the creation of an unadorned and unequivocal space of worship.

> You must perceive that this enlargement is made with all possible economy and prudence. Ostentation is not here blended with charity; the beneficence is not here squandered (as may sometimes be seen) in ornament and pomp; the curious artist has not here been permitted to exhibit his taste and skill at the poor penitents' expense; no vaulted domes or guilded ceilings, no swelling columns or sculptured capitals adorn this humble roof; no crowned or mitred canopies are erected to point out wealth and title to the gazing crowd. None here can pray in state. But all must kneel without distinction as partakers of the same impartial God.
> (Quoted in Peter, 1907, pp 18–20; Figure 70).

By the time Warburton, Whitelaw and Walsh wrote about it in 1818, the chapel at the Leeson Street Asylum had been extended again to accommodate a total of 700 people. Their description of both it and the Lock Penitentiary (Bethesda) chapel alludes to one of the reasons for its popularity: the opportunity for a middle-class congregation to share a space with a group of unseen *impures* whose presence, evinced by their 'pensive and sweet' voices, gave the service 'a peculiarly interesting solemnity'. Even here, in the austerity

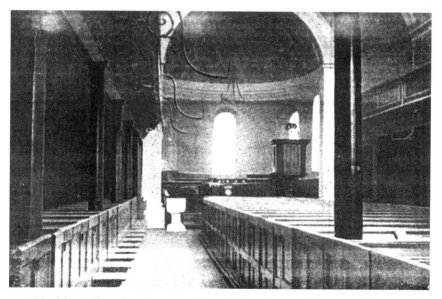

70 Magdalen Asylum chapel in Leeson Street in the early twentieth century. (Peter, 1907.)

of a chapel shorn of unnecessary excess to focus the mind purely on spiritual and moral matters, their words remain not a little suggestive, a quality which is shared by their passionate account of the Bethesda chapel.

> The chapel of the Bethesda is usually crowded during divine service, either because it is supposed the service is performed with more solemnity, the preaching more impressive, or the doctrine more pure. Perhaps the excellent uses to which the establishment is applied may attract many to this house of worship. They hear on one side the voice of the female penitent, and on the other, of the female orphan, joining in divine service; the first having past through the extremes of misery and vice, returning unchastened and reformed to the house of God; the second, as yet pure and unacquainted with sin and wretchedness, contrasted with their unhappy sisters and taking a solemn warning by their example. The impression of this is very affecting, and the voice of one penitent in particular has been long celebrated for its pensive sweetness.
> (Warburton, Whitelaw and Walsh, 1818, p. 775)

Denied a visual connection, ambiguities linger on within the aural and imaginative realms, an implication which is not diminished by the fact that David La Touche (III), regular client of Mrs Leeson's brothel, was treasurer of the Lock Penitentiary and held a pew at the Leeson Street Asylum where his wife was a member of the committee (Watson's *Almanack*, 1797).

Beyond the solemn female chanting of the chapel, however, both organizations were disciplinary institutions. The Leeson Street Asylum, complete with 'a code of laws for its internal government' (Curry, 1841, pp 248–9), required that on entry young women relinquished their former identities and assumed new ones. Here, penitents were forbidden to use their own names and instead were issued with a number, becoming known as Mrs One, Mrs Two, Mrs Three etc. (Luddy and Murphy (eds), 1990, p. 64). Strict control was also exercised over both space and time. Denny, who had previously presented a clock which chimed every twenty minutes to regulate the feeding of babies to the Foundling Hospital, had an hourglass placed in the middle of the dining table where the penitents could watch the sands run out as they ate or took their thirty minutes of exercise (Peters, 1905, p. 56). Despite being ostensibly designed specifically for young women abandoned after their 'first fall', the location of the asylum so close to St Stephen's Green suggests its remit also included extending a visual reminder of moral discipline to the

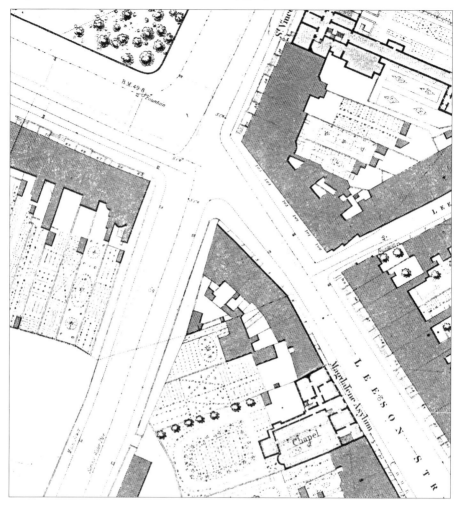

71 Leeson Street Magdalen Asylum near St Stephen's Green
(Ordnance Survey, 'five foot' plan, Sheet 28 (1847)).

public space outside the building and, perhaps especially, the more hardened streetwalkers and their clients who, according to contemporary sources, regularly stalked the Green (Lyons, 1995, p. xii; Figure 71).

Vice and the closure of the Pleasure Gardens

Prostitution in the eighteenth century was arranged in a social hierarchy which corresponded closely to the status of its clientele (Lyons, 1995, p. xi). At the zenith were courtesans and 'kept-women', the discrete and temporarily monogamous sexual companions of the rich and powerful. From there the practice descended into more commercial and explicit forms. While Leeson's establishments were high-class affairs accommodating an elite clientele, other, downmarket brothels serviced the lower classes. On the bottom rung, however, was the most visible and public, the common streetwalker. It was this last category which, according to Magee in the *Dublin Evening Post*, had, by 1797, reached epidemic proportions in certain parts of the city. In fact, the early concern for the control of the lower echelons of the practice, evinced by the establishment and location of the Leeson Street Asylum, intensified towards the end of the century. In 1792, John Fane, earl of Westmoreland and lord lieutenant (and, according to Leeson, illicit lover of Mrs Sinnot), decreed that the Lock Hospital be relocated from the suburbs of Donnybrook and established in the city, indicating a growing disquiet for the sanitary consequences of profligacy: venereal disease ('Boardroom Minute Book', 1792, Westmoreland Lock Hospital Records).

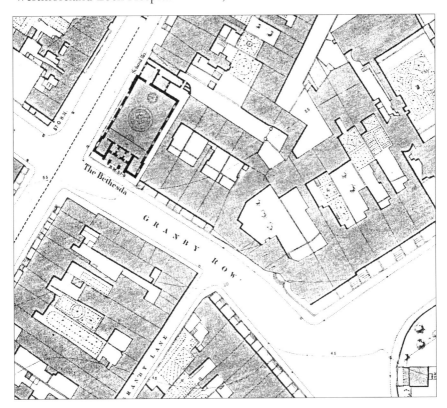

72 The Lock Penitentiary (Bethesda) near Rutland Square.
(Ordnance Survey 'five foot' plan, Sheet 8 (1847)).

Meanwhile, as the social profile of the pleasure gardens' clientele declined in the latter stages of the eighteenth century, sexual adventure in the vicinity tended to shift from more discrete dalliances, simultaneously obscured and accommodated by the heterogeneity of the gardens and the hospital, into more commercialized and visible forms. The first brothel in Great Britain Street had appeared by 1778. By 1796 there were at least two. From the description of Leeson, it seems the second of these was both successful and downmarket. 'Trench's Act' of 1784, therefore, can also be placed in the context of these developments. Similarly, the Lock Penitentiary (Bethesda chapel) established in 1794, just around the corner in Dorset Street, mirrors the Leeson Street asylum in providing a built manifestation of righteousness in an area linked with dubious morality (Figure 72).

The glittering mask of the Ascendancy's vision of Ireland as a discrete Protestant entity cracked irrevocably in the rebellion of 1798. Inspired by the French and American Revolutions, Wolfe Tone's rhetoric of the 'rights of man' regardless of whether 'Catholic, Protestant or Dissenter' confirmed the radical presence of some of those neglected by or excluded from the 'bungling, imperfect business' of 1782 (Tone, 1791). Fittingly, the events of 1798 also confirmed the demise of the pleasure gardens, Rotunda and Assembly Rooms as an elite leisure resort. For the duration of the upheaval collectively they were closed and the buildings converted temporarily into a government barracks. They reopened just in time for the Act of Union and the closure of the Irish Parliament. The landed aristocrats and members of parliament who had graced the site for decades would disappear forever.

In 1800, the site endured further ignominy at the hands of a group of moral crusaders. *The Association for the Discountenancing of Vice, and Promoting the Knowledge and Practice of the Christian Religion* was formed by three individuals in a house in Capel Street in October 1792. By 1795, the organization had a membership of five hundred which included the viceroy, Lord Fitzwilliam. Its *raison d'être* was simple:

> That the rapid progress which infidelity and immorality are making throughout the kingdom calls loudly on every individual of the clergy and laity who has at the heart the welfare of his country and the honour of his God, to exert all his powers to stem the baneful torrent.
> (Warburton, Whitelaw and Walsh, 1818, p. 886)

A series of duties were introduced to counteract moral decadence and encourage rectitude. Bibles were disseminated and a campaign launched to suppress licentious and obscene books which, 'were prime agents in the hands of infidelity to demoralize the people'. On at least one occasion a literary *auto-da-fé* was invoked, as 'they induced [a hawker] to render up his impure commodities, which were burned by their direction'. Other vices which caught their notice included gambling and intemperance, 'the consumption of spirituous liquors was … a pregnant source of immorality and misery'. Most pointed, however, was a critique on what essentially had been the New Pleasure Gardens' accepted *modus operandi* for over half a century.

> [T]o discourage and discountenance luxury, dissipation, and extravagance in the upper and middle classes, both male and female.
> (Warburton, Whitelaw and Walsh, 1818, p. 886)

Accordingly, the organization petitioned and succeeded in having the Sunday evening promenade, the most profitable event of the week, closed down because it was in 'violation of the Sabbath'. This censure, located at the very end-point of the eighteenth century, seems symptomatic of the emerging concern for the moral supervision and propagation of good behaviour popularly associated with the following epoch. The reality, however, was more complex. Other events and organizations were also conspiring to alter Dublin's moral profile. The billeting of troops in the Rotunda during the 1798 rebellion attracted an additional concentration of lower-class prostitutes and camp followers to the north-east sector of the city. In 1797, Sir Ralph Abercromby, Commander of Militia and Yeomanry, described his command as being 'in a state of licentiousness which must render it formidable to everyone but the enemy' (quoted in Foster, 1988, p. 227).

Spaces of empire

A militarized society

The 1790s in Ireland have been described as a decade of revolution, republicanism and ultimately reaction. The war with France, which began in 1793, soon became a titanic struggle for dominance, one which involved numbers of men, amounts of *matériel* and sums of money on an unprecedented scale. Consequently, the Irish budget, solvent before 1793, ran at an increasing loss for the rest of the decade as the conflict consumed nearly 78% of government expenditure (Bartlett and Jeffrey, eds, 1996, p. 247). The effects of the war when viewed against the potent spectre of the French revolution, effectively polarized politics in Ireland as shadowy insurgents groups emerged to seize the opportunity to ally themselves with England's enemy (Foster, 1988, pp 262–3). One such group, the United Irishmen counted amongst its figureheads the flamboyant Lord Edward FitzGerald who epitomized a proclivity amongst certain sections of the aristocracy, for the radical chic of all things Gallic and revolutionary. Accordingly, there was a growing sense of unease amongst the British executive in Dublin Castle concerning the double-threat of a French invasion aided and abetted by indigenous uprising. These fears were ultimately realized in the events of 1798, when the incursion of the French expeditionary force of General Humbert deep into the heart of the country in late summer, coincided with the last moments of the United Irish rebellion.

At the same time, the British war machine was demanding a constant re-supply of recruits for its campaigns. Thus, in the years between 1793 and 1815, intensive recruitment drives ensured that approximately one in five Irish adult males experienced military service. Moreover, the British government had been forced to reconsider its longstanding policy of entrusting Protestants alone with the defence of Ireland. The establishment of the largely Catholic Irish Militia, as well as other measures designed to adhere Catholic loyalties to the British Crown and entice Catholics, the most plentiful supply of men, into the Crown Forces, therefore, represented a radical departure. Meanwhile, fears of a union between the aims of the United Irishmen and the Catholic cause and the possibilities of a resultant armed rebellion, provoked the establishment of an almost entirely Protestant yeomanry as a counter-insurgent force in 1796.

Sectarian tensions aside, the consequences of this massive military build-up – Crown Forces in Ireland rose from 9,644 to 116,584 between January 1793 and January 1800 – was a period of unprecedented military involvement in affairs of state and military presence in everyday life. This was perhaps epitomised by the decision to appoint Charles, Earl Cornwallis as both lord lieutenant and commander-in-chief of the government forces in Ireland. Indeed, it was Cornwallis who, not only organised the speedy suppression of the 1798 rebellion but also 'seized the opportunity the crisis offered to put through a legislative union between Ireland and England' and dissolve the Irish Parliament (Bartlett in Bartlett and Jeffrey, 1996, pp 248–88). According to contemporary chroniclers Warburton, Whitelaw and Walsh, however, the convergence of military and civil society had other consequences – it created the conditions for a countrywide epidemic of immorality, profligacy and the proliferation of one specific type of disease.

> [I]t is one of the many evils naturally attendant on the present unparalleled state of Europe: large standing armies have unhappily become necessary for our protection; in every large town, nay, in every small village, troops are now quartered permanently; and that to this circumstance, the more extensive propagation of the venereal disease in the capital, and throughout every part of Ireland is to be attributed, the sick reports of the army afford irrefragable proofs; nor can it be concealed or denied, that an increased profligacy of manners amongst the lower order of females is distinctly to be traced to the same origin.
> (Warburton, Whitelaw and Walsh, 1818, p. 696)

Prostitution, venereal disease and the Westmoreland Lock Hospital, Dublin

Throughout the eighteenth and nineteenth centuries, venereal disease often featured in the list of conditions which precluded entry into most hospitals. In 1733, for example, Steeven's Hospital required, '[t]hat the patients admitted be the sick and wounded poor of all religions, labouring under curable distempers, neither venereal or infectious' (Governors' Meeting, July 1733, quoted in Croker King, 1785, p. 8). Similarly, the Lying-in Hospital – as evinced by their Admissions Card (see above, Figure 67) – still stipulated the non-admission of venereal patients as well as other 'contagious distempers' well into the nineteenth century.

While there may have been sound medical reasons for the non-admission of incurables and fever patients or even pregnant women, the exclusion of those with venereal disease appears to have been predicated purely on moral grounds. Indeed, even in the non-discriminating ethos of *ancien régime* hospitals, like the Hôtel Dieu in Paris, an exception was often made with those whose suffering had resulted from sexual misadventure (Quétel, 1990, p. 291). Elsewhere in France, the seventeenth-century Daughters of Charity stipulated that they 'should not take care of paupers suffering from venereal disease and that *femmes et filles de mauvaise vie* should be systematically excluded' (Jones in Finzsch and Jütte, 1996, p. 64). Meanwhile, in Protestant England, St Thomas's Hospital in London did accept venereal patients but

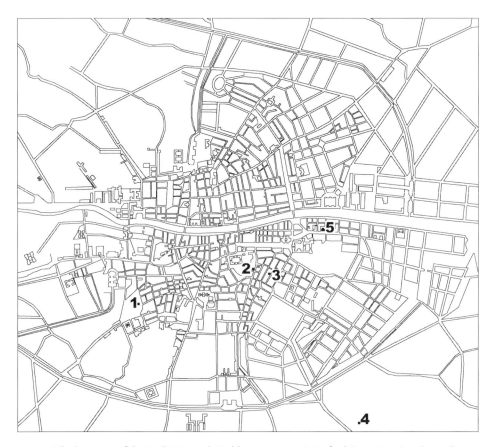

73 The locations of the Lock Hospital, Dublin, 1755–92: **1** Rainsford Street (1755), **2** George's Lane (in the vacated site of the Lying-in Hospital, 1758), **3** Clarendon Street, **4** Donnybrook (in the vacated site of the Buckingham Hospital, 1778), **5** Townsend Street (in the vacated site of the Hospital for Incurables, 1792). (Compiled by the author, based on Taylor, 1816.)

confined them to a series of irregularly shaped 'foul wards', situated in a side court, specifically reserved for the 'victims of a disease so degrading to humanity' (quoted in Thompson and Goldin, 1975, p. 84).

In Dublin, the Lock Hospital, established in 1755 (nine years after the founding of a similar institution in London) was one of the most peripatetic of the city's voluntary hospitals (Figure 73). Throughout its early years it drifted indiscriminately through a succession of appropriated properties whose location and characteristics reveal no obvious pattern or consistency: Rainsford Street was a small detached house on the fringes of the city and George's Lane was the vacated backland site of the former maternity hospital. This and the subsequent location in Clarendon Street (the exact site is unknown) were in the city centre. All were resolutely small-scale. After Clarendon Street, the hospital moved to the countryside where it languished in the unused Buckingham Smallpox Hospital, neglected even by its own consulting surgeons, 'who were reluctant to drive all the way to Donnybrook to assist the patients' (Watson's *Almanack*, 1794, p. 104).

In 1792, however, the hospital experienced a marked reversal of fortune. In June of the previous year, Arthur Wolfe, Lord Kilwarden and attorney general, informed the governors of the Hospital for Incurables that the government wished to exchange the Lock Hospital for their premises on Townsend Street because it 'required a substantial lock hospital near the centre of the city' (Watson's *Almanack*, 1794, p. 104). The decision was explained in more detail retrospectively in the board room minutes of the new hospital in 1800.

> In consequence of the Number of Poor of both Sexes in this city afflicted with Venereal Diseases whose situation called loudly for Relief, His Excellency the Earl of Westmoreland, the lord lieutenant was pleased in 1792, to desire the Opinion and Advice of Several Respectable Members of the College of Physicians and Surgeons as to the means most likely to check or alleviate the progress of this Disease, among the lower ranks of the People. The gentlemen who were consulted stated to His Excellency that, as the House of Industry was not adapted and the hospitals in the Metropolis were inadequate to the Reception of so numerous and increasing a class, it has in their opinion, become a Measure of Indispensable, Public Necessity to open an Extensive Hospital, for the Indiscriminate Admission and Accommodation of that Description of Patients who should be received without any Recommendation whatsoever.
> ('General Lock-hospital Board Room Minutes, 1792', hereafter 'Lock Minutes', 1800)

On 20 November 1792, the institution, now called the Westmoreland Lock Hospital, reopened on its new urban site with the admission of 120 patients. The name change, while honouring John Fane, earl of Westmoreland, lord lieutenant and sponsor of the move, also announced a corresponding shift in the administration of the hospital from an independent board of governors to one which was directly accountable to the executive at Dublin Castle. This indicated a substantial alteration in the significance of venereal disease. At a time of unprecedented danger to the sovereignty of the British Isles, the disease's potentially debilitating effect on a standing army made it increasingly a matter of national security. In turn, this military interest helped to accelerate a process of redefinition, not only of venereal disease but also of its cohort, illicit sexual activity in the form of prostitution, from being perceived as primarily religious and moral concerns into a situation where they were regarded as legitimate medical and scientific problems.

Outside Britain and Ireland this process was significantly more advanced. In France in 1778, for example, the military authorities introduced, for the first time, 'a proper campaign of prophylaxis for the armed forces' which included the compulsory admission of prostitutes to hospitals for examination and treatment (Quétel, 1990, p. 291). Towards the end of the century, other techniques emerged all over Europe to place prostitutes under surveillance and make the practice and its consequences more visible. By 1796, in Paris, prostitutes were obliged to make themselves known to the authorities by placing their names on an official register. Failure to do so resulted in their tracking down by a team of special agents. They were also subject to a series of spatial controls similar to those prescribed for Dublin by Magee in his 1797 harangue in the *Dublin Evening Post.* Forbidden to solicit in public streets, prostitutes were compelled to inhabit specific quarters of the city where they were kept under the control of the police as a distinct caste. Surveillance of the prostitute in urban space, however, was mirrored by the simultaneous surveillance of the prostitute's body. By 1798, those living in licensed brothels were required to submit themselves once a week for sanitary inspection and had to carry a card attesting to a clean bill of health, signed by the inspecting officer and stamped with the date. If found to be infected, they were immediately dispatched to Saint-Lazare Hospital for treatment (Bullough and Bullough, 1987, pp 188–90).

The figure of the prostitute, therefore, appears to stand at the vanguard of the process of increased medical intervention by State authorities into all aspects of public life which emanated from France during the last quarter of the eighteenth century and especially after 1791 (Foucault, 2000). The conceptual leap necessary to irrevocably shed the traditional moral prejudices attached to venereal disease and prostitution was, however, never completed. Indeed, many of the modern medical measures executed in Paris in the eighteenth and nineteenth centuries bore a marked resemblance to age-old techniques for dealing with objects of fear. Nowhere was this continuity between notionally objective science and superstition more evident than in the space of the hospital.

Constructed on the site of a leper-colony, throughout its history Saint-Lazare testified to the retributive and punitive results of transgression: from 1632 onwards it was a work-house; during the Reign of Terror it was an antechamber for the guillotine and afterwards a women's prison, before gradually being transformed into the 'prison-hospital of sinister repute' which was dreaded by prostitutes until its ultimate closure in 1940 (Quétel, 1990, p. 215). Its very name, moreover, evoked lingering associations with its original inhabitants. For Foucault, the leper provided an enduring metaphor for the exercise of irrational power over marginal bodies. In the Middle Ages, leprosy was the unique subject of a series of taboos and superstitions which, like the measures taken to regulate prostitution in Paris, manifested themselves in spatial prohibitions. Lepers were assigned discrete enclaves within the landscape downwind of towns and other settlements. They were forbidden to enter inns, churches, mills or bakehouses, to touch healthy people or eat with them or to wash in streams or public drinking fountains. Steps were also taken to ensure their identity was both continually made visible and unequivocally defined – they had to wear a certain uniform or manner of dress or carry a clapper or bell to warn of their approach. The anxiety that ambiguity could cause was expressed in a law which forbade them to 'walk in narrow paths at evening times' lest the diminished visibility produce an unexpected moment of proximity (Lee, 1996, p. 13). These prohibitions were borne out of a fear of contagion which was inextricably bound up with ideas of morality and religion. Contemporary perception of the disease often considered it a divine or diabolic intervention, punishment for an unseen iniquity committed by the victim (Foucault, 1993; Sumption, 1975, p. 78).

Like post-Revolutionary France, in Dublin, the perceptual shift necessary to transform venereal disease from pestilence into an objectively considered disease was fraught with and undermined by superstitious and moral associations. Indeed, even the generic term 'lock' hospital derived from the French *locques*, the bandages applied to lepers' sores (Papworth, ed., 1852–92, p. 83). It was first used to describe an institution at Southwark near London in 1452 where the 'Lock Lazar-House' subsequently became a venereal hospital. In Dublin, like at Saint-Lazare, Paris, this linguistic continuity was intensified: the Lock Hospital's new site at Townsend Street was loaded with historical connotations. In fact, the street had only been so-named since the vice-royalty of George, fourth Viscount Townsend, between 1767 and 1772 (McCready, 1892, p. 206). Hitherto, it had been known as Lazars (or Lazer's) Hill or by the colloquial but equally pejorative corruptions of Lazy, Lowzy or Lousy Hill. Its etymology lay in the establishment of the St James or Steyne Hospital in the vicinity in the twelfth century. This hospital, whose history remains shrouded in mystery, was apparently created to accommodate the roving bands of sick pilgrims who were on their way to, or returning from, Santiago de Compostella (Archdall, 1786; Haliday, 1884; *Irish Builder*, 15 August and 15 October 1896). The building subsequently vanished, leaving only the collective name of its inmates as proof of its existence. The geographic coincidence between the leper and the venereal victim in Dublin, however, was contingent on the presence of another group of intermediary outsiders, whose treatment also straddled the boundaries between superstition and medicine.

The Hospital for Incurables

Remote and hidden from the city by the bulk of Trinity College, Lazar's Hill shadowy associations with society's outsiders was re-emphasised in 1754 with the arrival, in the insalubrious vicinity of 'Pounder's Foundery', of the Hospital for Incurables (Figure 74). At first, such an institution appears to explicitly contradict the concept of a productive hospital discussed above in chapter 1. As has been shown, the curable/incurable boundary marked the key distinction in the divide, emerging in the latter part of the eighteenth century, between the *ancien régime* institution and the prototypical modern, medical hospital. Indeed, even as early as 1733, the regulations of Steeven's Hospital in common with other voluntary hospitals in Dublin was stipulating the exclusion of those whose affliction was beyond the reach of medical and surgical treatment: 'in case a Patient shall be found, in the process of time incurable, then to be discharged' (Governors' Meeting, July 1733, quoted in Croker King, 1785, p. 8).

The interpretation of 'incurable', in the context of the eponymous hospital, however, does not quite resonate with the modern definition of the word. In 1745, Watson's *Almanack* published its first notice of the hospital which not only described its founding by a Charitable Musical Society in 1743 (the

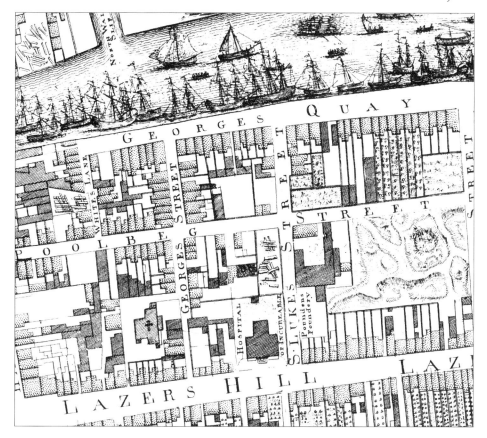

74 The Hospital for Incurables on Lazers Hill. (John Rocque, *Exact Survey*, 1756.)

president of which was Lord Mornington), but also revealed the two interlinking aspects of its mission.

> The Wretched are here maintained and their Infirmities palliated, and the Publick in a great measure freed from those disagreeable sights, so frequently heretofore met with in our streets.
>
> (Watson's *Almanack*, 1745)

When, in 1748, the hospital made an appeal in the same publication for more funds, the emphasis had shifted slightly. To address a financial shortfall, the governors resolved to only admit 'those miserable objects who are offensive to sight' (Watson's *Almanack*, 1748). The definition of incurable used by the hospital, therefore, appears to have been predicated as much on aesthetic criteria – deformity and disability – as it was on the modern sense of a terminal illness. Moreover, the concern for the 'incurables' themselves seems secondary to a desire to have them removed from the streets. The notice in the Watson's *Almanack* of 1748 also requested that 'Ministers and Churchwardens of each parish' send their Beadle with such persons to the Hospital'. This service was rewarded by half a guinea paid to the Beadle 'after the admission of such objects has been confirmed'. In fact, this aesthetic policy was reiterated in print annually for the next twenty-five years. Moreover, a text published in 1865, by Dr Cheyne Brady, a member of the committee of the hospital, implies that such measures enjoyed an enduring quasi-medical legitimacy.

> Although our streets are now free from the offensive and dangerous practice of the exposure of frightful cases of disease, yet living memory can recall the time when the senses were wont to be disgusted by the sight of cripples and other loathsome objects, who were carried to a frequented thoroughfare, and there exposed to excite the compassion of passers-by.
>
> (Brady, 1865, p. 5)

Brady's demarcation of the sight of 'cripples and loathsome objects' as dangerous, suggests a continuation in the belief of 'contamination by sight' (Stafford, 1993, p. 306). This superstition held that visual phenomena could cause actual bodily harm, especially it seems, to vulnerable females, an eventuality which Warburton, Whitelaw and Walsh allude to in their description of incurables in Dublin who, 'by being exposed in the streets, exhibited objects not only offensive to humanity, but dangerous to delicate and pregnant females' (1818, p. 728). The belief was certainly persistent and its reiteration in the *Irish Builder* in 1897, which described vagrants 'with the most offensive sores, or such deformities, disgusting to all and dangerous in their efforts to the beholders', suggests its logic may have even continued into the twentieth century.

In the nebulous zone between superstition and primitive medical theory, therefore, the Hospital for Incurables perhaps had some of the active and progressive attributes of a modern hospital. Indeed, it is important to remember that, in the days before X-ray and other imaging techniques, diseases only existed when they became manifest on the skin. It has been suggested that this contributed to the importance, during the eighteenth-century Enlightenment, of 'an aesthetic of immaculateness' which fostered the creation of a whole

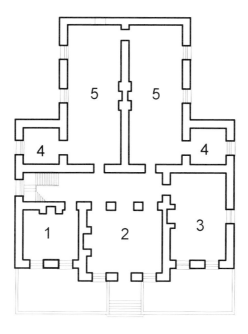

75 Ground floor plan of the Hospital for Incurables, 1753–92: **1** consultants' apartment; **2** entrance hall; **3** boardroom; **4** nurses' rooms; **5** wards. (Drawn by author, based on drawings in the Murray Collection, Irish Architectural Archive.)

series of cosmetics to produce, on the individual, an unblemished public face (Stafford, 1993, p. 283). A similar process can be perceived as operating on the surface of the city of Dublin. Created just as the upper classes were vacating the unsanitary and heterogeneous old town for the socially homogeneous new suburbs, the Hospital for Incurables intersected a moment where ideologies of aesthetics and health merged within the public realm. The suburbs, a landscape of wide streets and ordered façades, produced an increased visibility which had been impossible in the narrow winding streets of the old town. On such a surface, the presence of blemish and disease became more starkly and unambiguously evident, simultaneously producing new anxieties and the need for new measures to exclude or conceal them.

The architect of the Hospital for Incurables remains in dispute. Some have suggested that it resembles the work of George Semple, while others liken it to the Palladian style of Richard Cassels or his protégé John Ensor (Craig, 1992, p. 168). The building, like Cassel's Lying-in Hospital or Semple's St Patrick's Lunatic Asylum, was based on a Palladian villa. Similar to St Patrick's, however, the hierarchy of space in its interior displayed an unequivocal front-to-back relationship. Perhaps understandably in a hospital whose function was to contain and conceal the offensive sights removed from the street, most, if not all of the patients inhabited ward spaces located at the rear of the building. Of the six wards, the four largest were arranged in a perpendicular return at the back of the house (two above two), flanked by nurses' rooms, with the remaining smaller pair located in the attic storey, perhaps also at the rear. The basement contained the usual sundry services of laundries, kitchens etc., while the elevated ground floor on the street side contained the more sumptuous spaces of the governors' board-room, the entrance hall and the consultants' apartment (Figure 75).

Like a cosmetic mask which attempts to 'obliterate all existential signs' on the face of its wearer (Stafford, 1993, p. 283), at first, the implacable façade of the Hospital for Incurables, 'built in mountain granite and of the Doric Order, and in a style plain, solid and durable' (Warburton, Whitelaw and Walsh, 1818, p. 696), offered an ordered and beautiful countenance to the public realm (Figure 76). In a short space of time, however, even this superficial harmony was perturbed. Like so many other eighteenth-century hospitals in Dublin, the concern for the creation of a palatial building was not matched by a concern for its subsequent organization and administration. Or, as Warburton, Whitelaw and Walsh (1818, p. 729) put it, 'the zeal and ability evinced in [the] erection [of the Hospital for Incurables] were not continued for its support and for several years this excellent charity languished in an obscure and negligent manner'. Perhaps inevitably, the first victims were the patients. By 1790, only two of the wards were occupied 'by a few of both sexes, who were seldom supplied with clothes, and exhibited an appearance equally squalid and offensive'. Shortly after, since the majority of the house was empty, the governors decided to admit incurable inmates transferred from the House of Industry, a decision which was described as unfortunate:

> The class of patients sent from the House of Industry were necessarily of the lowest description; they brought with them all the vicious and immoral practices of early habits and soon introduced among the established patients of the house … their own habits and propensities. In a short time the hopeless irregularities and profligacy of the house induced the governors to render up the whole establishment to the governors of the House of Industry, from a despair of managing it as they intended, [although] happily the measure was abandoned.
> (Warburton, Whitelaw and Walsh, 1818, p. 729)

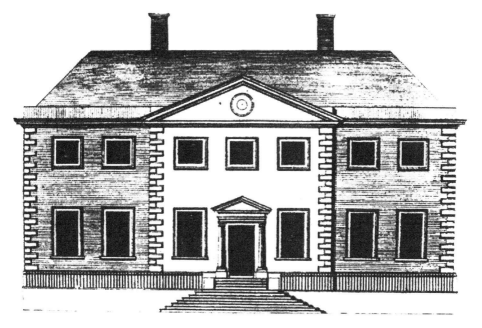

76 Hospital for Incurables, Lazers Hill. (engraving after J. Aheron, 1762.)

John Howard's short but condemning account of the hospital published in 1791 in his celebrated *Account of the principle Lazarettos of Europe* implies the disorder and neglect of the wards at the rear had managed to manifest itself throughout the building and perhaps even on its public face: 'Both outside and inside dirty:- the rooms are offensive:- no rules:- no diet table:- the housekeeper is in the country. The Mistresses of such houses should never be permitted to be absent' (Howard, 1791, p. 38).

From house to machine: Richard Johnston and the Westmoreland Lock Hospital

In June 1792, immediately after the city's incurables had been banished to the hinterland of Donnybrook, a programme of building works began on their former abode. The government's aspiration to create 300 new beds for male and female venereal patients required the construction of new wards at the hospital. In an ironic reversal, Richard Johnston, architect of the Assembly Rooms, haunt of the upper class libertine, was commissioned to construct the State's response to the 'profligacy of the lower orders' (Warburton, Whitelaw and Walsh, 1818, p. 696). While nothing physical is left of the Westmoreland

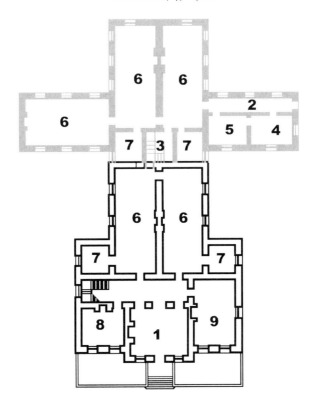

77 Ground floor plan of the Westmoreland Lock Hospital, Townsend Street, showing additions by Richard Johnston, 1792: **1** main entrance; **2** patients' entrance; **3** central staircase; **4** apothecary's shop; **5** surgery; **6** wards; **7** nurses' rooms; **8** consultant's apartment; **9** boardroom. (Drawn by author, based on drawings in the Murray Collection, Irish Architectural Archive.)

Lock Hospital, the few remaining plans in existence (contained in the Murray Collection in the Irish Architectural Archive) suggest Johnston's response to such an emphatically joyless brief was as austere and utilitarian as the Assembly Rooms were flamboyant and magnificent. Leaving the Palladian frontage well alone, the architect added an inverted T-shaped extension to the rear, effectively consolidating the front to back relationship and splitting the building into two discrete zones, each with a separate entrance. As before, consultants and governors entered through the grand Doric door piece on the building's front façade. Patients, on the other hand, were now admitted at the rear of the building from the side through an entrance located around the corner on Luke Street, in the eastern branch of the 'T'. Here, one passed by a type of out-patients' department consisting of an apothecary's shop and surgery before entering through a door into a ward, from where one could access a central staircase. This vertical circulation core, lit by a glass roof lantern, not only serviced the extension but also connected the wards located in the older part of the hospital. In plan, it resembles a hub around which a cruciform of ward space is arrayed, an arrangement which hints at the presence of medical or scientific principles in the genesis of the design (Figure 77).

The cruciform plan had its origins in the long medieval infirmary hall which contained at its end-point an altar or shrine. In the religious ether of the *ancien régime* hospital, the altar, signifier of a grace and succour beyond the boundaries of medicine, was designed to be seen by all. Its position at the intersection of two or more wards, like in Filarette's double-cross plan *Ospedale Maggiore* (*c.*1465) (Figure 78), meant it could simultaneously serve a series of separate spaces. According to Foucault and others, during the Enlightenment's disenchantment of the world, this visibility was effectively inverted to become the mechanism of a more material type of control. In other words, divine omnipotence was replaced by clinical, or indeed reformatory, surveillance (Foucault 1993, Markus, 1993, pp 107–8). The central hub – through which everyone must pass – is in a position to observe everything while each spoke radiating from it accommodates the medically prescribed isolation of a single class of patient.

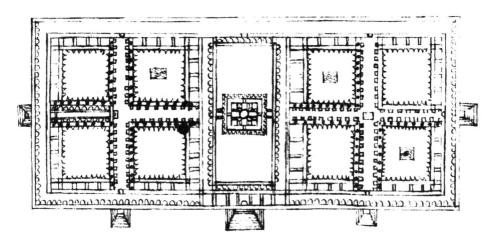

78 *Ospedale Maggiore*, Milan. (Filarette, *c.*1465.)

In Johnston's extension to the Lock Hospital, the circulation core, combined with two strategically positioned 'Nurses' Rooms', performed a similar function, controlling movement between the branches of the cruciform and thus segregating the patients into discrete zones. There are, however, compromises and inefficiencies which for the most part probably arose because the intervention was appended to an existing building. The central circulation core as a site of surveillance only really addresses the wards in the extension. Those in the older part of the building are watched by another two 'Nurses' Rooms' located in the zone between the front and back of the house. Furthermore, access to the central staircase from the street is through a ward which effectively short-circuits the isolation of the patients held there. Johnston's extension, however, also contained one other 'scientific' or 'medical' property. The two wards in the western branch of the 'T' (on ground and first floor level), as well as the ward above the apothecary and surgery in its eastern branch, all enjoyed cross ventilation.

This principle, so valued by Edward Foster in his 1768 treatise, was a key factor, along with the provision of isolation, in the development of the pavilion-ward plan, perhaps the ultimate manifestation of the belief that architecture could actually cure. Notwithstanding Foster's text and others like it, a positivistic faith in the medicinal potential of hospital buildings was only really consolidated in the wake of the destruction by fire of the Hôtel Dieu, the great rambling icon of *ancien régime* charity in 1772 (Middleton, 1993–94, p. 17). In the series of mostly unexecuted proposals for its replacement, alongside a whole range of new radial and circular forms, we find a pavilion scheme. It was the scientist-designer of this project, Jean-Baptiste Le Roy, who first uttered the memorable statement that, 'a ward is, as it were, a machine for treating the sick' (quoted in Pevsner, 1976, p. 151).

The pavilion's resurgence in mid-nineteenth-century Britain, to become, for about a century, the dominant ward form, owed much to its chief supporters' (most conspicuous among them were George Godwin and Florence Nightingale) unswerving, if misguided belief in the miasmatic theory of infection, that is, that disease is borne out of foul, fetid air (Thompson and Goldin, 1975, p. 118). According to this theory, the naturally (as opposed to mechanically) cross-ventilated pavilion standing in isolation was uniquely positioned to expel tainted atmospheres and thus prohibit the spread of disease. At the beginning of the nineteenth century in Dublin, the principles of cross-ventilation can be seen in the buildings constructed to deal with the city-wide emergency of a fever epidemic. The Cork Street Fever Hospital, for example, was built in 1801 as a response to a report carried out by T.A. Murray which highlighted the apparent problem of noxious miasma in the poorer areas of the city (Murray, 1801, p. 2; Figure 79). Accordingly, the building was

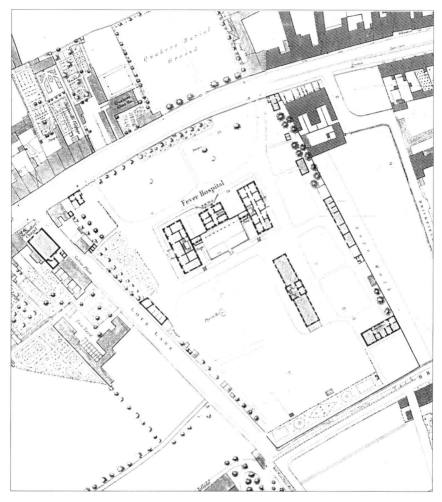

79 Plan of Cork Street Fever Hospital (1801) showing the isolated pavilion layout. (Ordnance Survey 'five-foot' plan, Sheets 25 and 26; 1847.)

designed and built as three linked pavilions under the close scrutiny of medical consultants, Dr Currie of Liverpool and Dr Percival and Beardsley of Manchester. Two years later in 1803, the Hardwicke Fever Hospital was also rebuilt under similar medical supervision.

In 1792, however, when the Westmoreland Lock Hospital extension was being constructed, only one other hospital in Dublin contained cross-ventilated wards: the Royal Military Infirmary, designed by James Gandon in 1786. Notwithstanding the building's symbolic function as a counterpart to the Royal Hospital Kilmainham in framing the city from the western

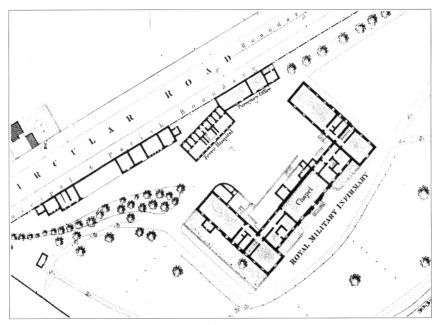

80 Plan of the Royal Military Infirmary, 1786.
(Ordnance Survey 'five-foot' plan, Sheet 12; 1847.)

approaches, it has been suggested that a great deal more planning in terms of medical needs went into its design than in any previous Dublin hospital. The building was formed in an H-plan shape with the ward space arranged in the two wings, separated from each other by an administration block (which also contained at least one ward). The six wards (three on each wing) at the rear end of the wings furthest from the central block are all fully cross-ventilated, whereas the six at the front enjoy partial cross-ventilation (Figure 80). Moreover and unusually for the time, the wards were designed for specific purposes and were strictly divided between medical and surgical patients with a separate, although curiously not cross-ventilated, pavilion for those suffering from fever (Casey in O'Brien and Crookshank, eds, 1984, p. 234).

To find such scientific rigour in a military hospital is no surprise. Issues of national security were often at the forefront of instigating new measures to preserve health. Compelled to provide medical care lest their charges die or desert, naval and military authorities in the eighteenth century often took a much more innovatory and experimental approach to the design of hospitals than their civil counterparts (Forty in King, ed., 1980, p. 66). Indeed, a version of Le Roy's pavilion arrangement had previously been used in the design for the Naval Hospital at Stonehouse near Plymouth, 1756–64.

Meanwhile in eighteenth-century France, military hospitals were able to follow an overtly functional orientation unencumbered, for the most part, by non-medical influences such as religious dogma, or indeed, the caprices of patrons and benefactors. A disciplined and hierarchically organized body of patients also contributed to an unfettered application of medical theory and experimentation. As well as being a site of innovation for environmental medicine such as ventilation, fumigation, hygiene, etc., military hospitals were also particularly suitable for clinical trials of new forms of medication and especially those relating to venereal disease (Jones in Finzsch and Jütte, eds, 1996, pp 68–9). This then begins to explain the medically progressive form of the Westmoreland Lock Hospital extension. Indeed, the institution's relocation to Townsend Street in 1792, coincided with the appointment of a new 'Board of Directors'.

> President College of Physicians, Vice President College of Physicians, Physician General, State Physician, President College of Surgeons, Vice-President College of Surgeons, Surgeon General, Surgeon to the King's Military Infirmary, Surgeon to the Royal Hospital, Kilmainham, State Surgeon, Professor of Surgery to the College of Physicians, Surgeon to the Police.
>
> (Watson's *Almanack,* 1794)

The overt military and medical profile (Physician and Surgeon General were Army commissions) of the Westmoreland Lock Hospital becomes more apparent when compared with the lists of governors of some other contemporary Dublin hospitals (or indeed, the London Lock Hospital, whose board between 1781 and 1837 was apparently dominated by the evangelical movement [Williams, 1988, pp 49–59]). We already know of the burgeoning board at the Lying-in Hospital, which by 1794 boasted a massive 58 members, but contained just two physicians and one surgeon (Watson's *Almanack*, 1794). Both Steeven's and St Patrick's had similar lists, comprised for the most part, of a mixture of peers of the realm, politicians, clergymen and legal figures, with a smattering of medics and surgeons. The board of Steeven's Hospital, for example, consisted of the following:

> Lord Primate, Lord Chancellor, Lord Archbishop Dublin, Chancellor of the Exchequer, Lord Chief Justice of the King's Bench, Lord Chief Justice of Common Pleas, Lord Chief Baron Exchequer, Dean of Christchurch, Dean of St Patrick's, Provost of Trinity College, Surgeon General, Thomas

Cobbe Esq., Henry, Viscount Palmerston, John Whitelaw, Esq., Joseph Henry Esq., J. Leigh, Esq., Treasurer, John Rochford, Sir Benjamin Chapman, Dr Clement Archer, Dr William Harvey, Rt Hon. James Cuffe, Samuel Croker King, Revd Dean Hastings.

(Watson's *Almanack*, 1794)

Liberated from the influence of non-medical governors, the Westmoreland Lock Hospital was also largely relieved of the necessity of raising and soliciting funds. It was financed directly by an annual parliamentary grant which, between 1797 and 1800, was paid at a rate of £4,600 net and was increased to £7,227 in 1803 ('Report to the Chancellor of the Exchequer' cited in 'Lock Minutes', October 1800 and December 1803). The architect Richard Johnston's rational and utilitarian extension took place, therefore, in the context of a similarly rationalized governing body and funding strategy. The functional clarity posited by the closer affiliation of medicine, administration and architectural form, if ever entirely fulfilled, was not enduring.

Disease, morality and further extensions at the Lock Hospital

[T]he chastity of the Irish female character in every class of life, has long been a subject of merited eulogy. Ireland, happily not far advanced in that progress of refinement which depraves the morals, while it gives a false polish to the manners, retained her primitive simplicity – the upper classes undisgraced by public scandal, and the lower undebauched by private profligacy. Dublin was, and perhaps still is, in that respect, the least vicious metropolis in Europe.

(Warburton, Whitelaw and Walsh, 1818, p. 696)

Warburton, Whitelaw and Walsh's tribute to the collective sexual purity of the Irish nation and indeed, its capital city, is largely contradicted by the experiences of its metropolitan venereal hospital. Between its opening on 20 November 1792 and 31 October 1793, 867 patients were discharged from the hospital and 1124 'received advice and medicines' ('Lock Minutes', February 1794). In March 1794, a letter from the board of directors to Westmoreland stated the 'additional buildings' (that is, Johnston's extension) were nearly complete, which would bring the capacity of the hospital to 300 beds, supplementing the existing situation of 100 male beds and 72 female beds. The letter added that women were turning up to apply for entry on a daily basis (Letter to Westmoreland cited in 'Lock Minutes', 4 March 1794).

By January 1795, the board were of the opinion that if the hospital was twice as large it would still be 'inadequate to the applications made for Admission'. Moreover, despite the professional profile of the governors, accusations were levelled by the Speaker of the House of Commons concerning partiality in the admissions procedure. Accordingly, it was resolved that 'Patients labouring under the most urgent and dangerous symptoms shall have the preference, when Beds become vacated' ('Lock Minutes', March 1795). There were, however, other problems concerning staffing. In 1795, the directors noted a high level of absenteeism amongst the consultants, forcing them to take the unusual step of resolving to pay an annual stipend, of £183 10s. 0d. for senior consultants and £50 for junior officers. Meanwhile in 1797, problems concerning patient admissions resurfaced, albeit in a slightly different form.

> Whereas it appears to the Board that Persons have been admitted into the Hospital having Fevers of an infectious kind accompanied by *lues venereal*, by which great and manifest injury has been done to other Patients, by introducing contagion in the House. It is therefore resolved that in future no Person whatever to be admitted into the Hospital who has any Fever which may be of an Infectious kind and this Resolution be notified to the senior Surgeon.
>
> ('Lock Minutes', October 1797)

The episode perhaps underlined the value of segregation and isolation in preventing the spread of disease. Segregation in a hospital designed to accommodate victims of a single malady, however, did not necessarily require the minute levels of differentiation posited by the pavilion plan or the radial schemes of large European institutions. While by 1800, there was a 'married women's ward' – perhaps indicating a distinction on moral grounds between profligates and innocent victims – and by 1805 the provision of convalescent wards had been proposed ('Lock Minutes', August 1800 and December 1805), the main focus of medical segregation in a lock hospital was presumably the prohibition of the activities which had put the patients there in the first place. Every modern institution and hospital operated the very basic spatial division between its male and female occupants, but in a hospital designed to cure the results of sexual activity this distinction assumed an extra urgency. Internal discipline and spatial segregation, however, proved to be inefficient when dealing with external agents, as revealed in the minutes from November 1801.

> It having been reported … that the Indulgence heretofore extended to Strangers in permitting them to visit their Friends on Wednesday from one to three o'clock has been attended with great Irregularity … and has produced serious bad effects. Ordered, that from henceforward … that no stranger be admitted in time to come into any of the wards without the steward's permission, or by producing an order to that effect written and assigned by one of the senior surgeons, an Indulgence which, for the state of preserving Quiet and Regularity in the Hospital, the Governors expect will never be granted by them without very urgent cause.
>
> ('Lock Minutes', November 1801)

By September 1804, however, even internal divisions between the hospital's male and female zones appear to have become porous, compelling the governors to introduce new measures to ensure that decency and decorum prevailed.

> Ordered that the senior Surgeons be authorised to make Alterations in the Hospital as may be necessary so as completely to make a separation between the Male and Female Patients and they are also further requested to point out and have fitted up a Military Guard to be established at the Hospital in the Future.
>
> ('Lock Minutes', September 1804)

The most obvious place for the split to happen was between Richard Johnston's extension and the older part of the hospital where movement was most controlled. An undated drawing entitled 'Sketch Design' shows a 'Guard Room' located in the eastern room of the central section of 'T'. From here you could watch the entry from the street through the apothecary's wing. The drawing, however, also shows a similar space located in the main entrance hall in the front section of the house. In December 1805, after a visit to the hospital, Hardwick, the incumbent lord lieutenant, suggested that the addition of two wards for convalescents would benefit the institution. It was subsequently proposed by the committee that these would fill 'the portion of ground on each side of the hospital'. The architect, Francis Johnston, younger brother of Richard, was asked to prepare an estimate for the costs of such a development and was subsequently commissioned to prepare plans for a scheme. In May 1806, his proposal encompassing two pavilions at the front of the building was approved.

Described by Maurice Craig as 'after Gandon, the greatest name in Irish architecture' (1992, p. 280), Francis Johnston was made Architect of the Board of Works and Civic Buildings in 1805, an appointment which may have been prompted by the alterations the architect made to the Foundling Hospital beginning in 1798. There, faced with an *ancien régime* institution, Johnston attempted to recast it as a modern instrument of reform by rationalising its plan to allow, like his elder brother Richard's extension at the Lock Hospital, the techniques of observation, classification and segregation to define and organise the building's interior space (Campbell, 1998, p. 42).

It is difficult to know, however, precisely what Johnston junior envisaged for the interior of the Lock Hospital or, indeed, what was actually carried out. A pen, ink and watercolour drawing of the ground floor plan, much marked with pencil corrections and notes, shows the introduction of a peripheral circulation system of two corridors linking the front pavilions with his brother's extension at the rear. This may have been an attempt, prompted by the governors' minutes of September 1804, to find a new way of dividing the building (this time longitudinally) into two discrete and isolated male and female zones (Figure 81). Whether executed or not remains unknown, but certainly the old problem caused by external visitors resurfaced in 1819 when 'much inconveniences and confusions had arisen from the custom of persons being allowed to indiscriminately visit patients once a week' ('Lock Minutes', March, 1819).

More intriguingly, Johnston's double corridor plan appears to deny the entry of fresh air to the two central wards on the ground floor of the older part of the house. But, while seeming to contradict the contemporary value placed on ventilation, it was perhaps not such an obvious error. The treatment of syphilis often involved the inhalation of mercury vapours (to provoke salivating) in specially adapted 'fluxing rooms' where ventilation was often not deemed necessary or even desirable. However, frequent references in the patient registers during the 1820s, to patients leaving the institution, because 'the hospital air [was] prejudice to her convalescence' or simply 'for air', suggest that acute problems were created in the building's atmospheric conditions ('General Register of Patients, 1816–21,' Westmoreland Lock Hospital Records). This is corroborated by Warburton, Whitelaw and Walsh who describe an environment heavily infused with the side-effects of fluxing:

> It being very desirable that one or two wards always be kept empty in a state of cleansing and purification, to admit the removal of patients in succession from a close and heated atmosphere, to breath pure air: and this provision seems to be the more necessary as some of the apartments in the old part of the house, which contain 17 or 18 beds,

have no ventilators, and are so filled with a mercurial atmosphere, as to produce a premature spitting, which by no means contributes to the cure of venereal disease.

(Warburton, Whitelaw and Walsh, 1818, p. 696)

Another 'Convalescent Ward', presumably for the type of patients Warburton, Whitelaw and Walsh describe, is noted in Francis Johnston's plan. It is not, however, located in the new wings, but rather on the upper storey of the western branch of his brother Richard Johnston's 'T' extension: i.e. in a cross ventilated ward. Other rooms in the 'T', however, have also been noted on the drawing as having new functions: below the 'Convalescent Ward' is the 'Laundry Dormitory' accompanying the adjacent 'Drying Room' and 'Laundry'. The two Nurses' Rooms are now a 'Porter's Kitchen' and the

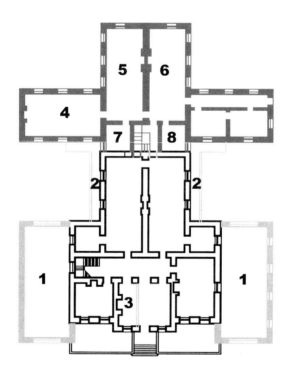

81 Ground Floor Plan of the Westmoreland Lock Hospital, showing alterations and additions by Francis Johnston (in light grey) in the early nineteenth century: **1** front pavilion wards; **2** corridors; **3** porter's room; **4** 'Laundry Dormitory' with convalescent ward above; **5** 'Drying Room'; **6** Laundry; **7** Laundry Kitchen; **8** Porter's Kitchen.
(Drawn by author based on drawings in the Murray Collection, Irish Architectural Archive.)

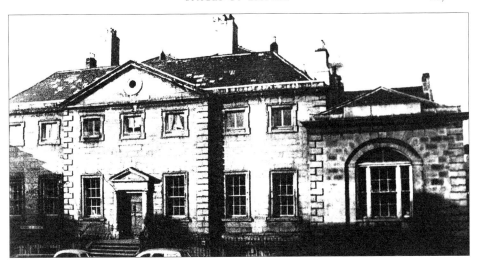

82 View of the Westmoreland Lock Hospital showing the new wing by Francis Johnston. (Mid-twentieth-century photograph, Irish Architectural Archive.)

'Laundry Kitchen'. With the possible exception of the 'Laundry Dormitory', buried at the furthest point from the street, Richard Johnston's extension, complete with the apothecary's shop and surgery now seems much more of a public zone and certainly not designed for the medical treatment of in-patients.

Moral management at the Lock Hospital

The presence of the laundry prefigures a major alteration in the hospital's *modus operandum*. In 1820, the institution closed its doors to male patients, reduced its number of beds to 150, half the original number, and became the exclusive domain of female venereal victims (Wright, 1825, pp 215–16). Simultaneously, the 'Board of Directors' was dissolved and replaced with a new 'Board of Governors', appointed by the lord lieutenant on 4 March 1820. It comprised of the following:

> Dean of St Patrick, Archdeacon of Dublin, Physician General, Surgeon General, Revd James Dunn, Paulus Æm Singer, John D. La Touche, Admiral Oliver, Major Woodward, William Disney.
>
> (Watson's *Almanack*, 1821)

While the committee is still well-represented by military, and to a lesser extent medical figures, its altered composition signals the end of twenty-eight years of undiluted medical and military administration. A number of underlying conditions may have influenced these changes. Firstly and perhaps most significantly, since the Battle of Waterloo the period of military crisis had ended. Accordingly, military presence in everyday life had greatly diminished – in the years immediately following 1815, for example, the standing army in Ireland halved in size (Spiers in Bartlett and Jeffrey, 1996, p. 335). No longer in a state of emergency and with a fifty per cent reduction in the army's capacity, State expenditure on the Lock Hospital at the same rate as before was no longer justifiable. On 23 August 1819, six months before the changes to the hospital took effect, the board room minutes record that the lord lieutenant proposed a significant reduction in the government grant to the hospital and had requested the directors to submit a statement of the institution's financial affairs to the executive at Dublin Castle. There were also sound medical reasons for the move. As has been shown, isolation of different patient groups was always considered desirable to prevent the spread of contagion. The hospital's minute books, however, testify to the building's periodic failure in prohibiting what were called 'irregularities' between male and female patients. The absolute separation of the sexes by locating them in different buildings, and indeed, different areas of the city, would seem to ensure that sexual misconduct between patients became more improbable, if not impossible.

However, the transformation of Dublin's only venereal hospital, from one accommodating diseased paupers of both sexes into a female only institution also seems symptomatic of a process which has recently been described as the 'feminisation of venereal disease' (Spongberg, 1997). This trend, which first emerged in late eighteenth-century medical discourse, posited the female body not only as the principal vector of the disease, but also its source. In the course of the nineteenth century, the scope of this misconception narrowed to focus more and more exclusively on the body of the prostitute, the iconic figure of extra-marital female sexuality. A hospital report published in Dublin, suggests that by 1818, a large proportion of female patients at the Westmoreland Lock Hospital were, in fact, prostitutes. It also, however, hints at a quasi-anatomical explanation for the growing association between their bodies and venereal disease: the apparent invisibility of the disorder on the female genitals in its initial stages, which, when combined with a professional promiscuity, created a fecund avenue of disease transmission.

> The Surgeon of the Westmoreland Lock Hospital have been long acquainted with the fact, that a morbid stage of the female genitals may

exist for several months without preventing male intercourse; and that thus affected, unfortunate prostitutes continue their wretched occupation until their complaints have proceeded to an extent which compels them to seek for relief.
(Todd in *Dublin Hospital Reports*, 1818, p. 185)

In fact, the anxieties caused by the ambiguous identity of those infected with venereal disease were to re-surface later in the century in a piece of parliamentary legislation. Beginning in 1864, and rather like the regulations established in Paris in the 1790s, the military-inspired Contagious Diseases Acts (CDAs), 1864, 1866, and 1869, prescribed the registration and intimate medical scrutiny (often with the dreaded *speculum*) of prostitutes in a series of garrison and naval towns throughout the British Isles. In Ireland, Cork, Queenstown (modernday Cobh) and Kildare/the Curragh were subject to the legislation while, perhaps curiously, Dublin was not. Notionally an objective and rational medical response to the proliferation of venereal disease and its incapacitating effect on the defence forces, the Contagious Diseases Acts contained an inherent double standard: the medical inspections of women were not extended to men. Moreover, in the attempt to determine the identity of prostitutes, working-class women of all descriptions often became the subject of suspicion or even forcible examination. These abuses were perhaps symptomatic of an ambiguous definition of prostitution which was borne out of middle-class preconceptions of the sexual habits of the working classes. It is exemplified here by the words of the reformer Henry Mayhew, first published in 1862, who suggested that 'literally every woman who yields to her passion and loses her virtue is a prostitute' (1862, p. 217).

When it was proposed to extend the Contagious Diseases Acts to civilian towns and cities, a series of campaigns against the legislation was organized, resulting in a huge moral backlash and public furore (Walkowitz, 1980, 1992; McHugh, 1980; Bullough and Bullough, 1987). Of all the barrages of argument and counter-argument between those for and against the acts – from prototypical feminists reacting angrily to the gender bias, evangelical crusaders campaigning against sin and immorality of all kinds, to pragmatically minded medical or military officers who saw inspection and regulation as the only reasonable course of action – one of the most salient moralistic arguments was that the medical model of prostitution did not actually cure the problem. Instead, according to the moralists, it posited an implicit tolerance and acceptance of illicit sexual activity: while attempting to physically cure the body, it made no correlative attempt on the behaviour which had led to disease in the first place. The Contagious Diseases Acts, for example, were not intended to suppress prostitution, *per se*, but rather, 'make the women who practice it less diseased, or as little diseased as may be, and therefore to make prostitution less injurious to mankind' (House of Commons Select Committee on the Administration, Operation and Effects of the Contagious Diseases Acts, 1866–9). Therein, lay one of the scheme's most potent criticisms, as evinced by this moral campaigner (writing in about 1870) who considered 'hospitals for prostitutes as elements in a machinery ... for giving an artificial security to promiscuous fornication' (quoted in Acton, 1870, p. 236). Others concurred, considering the CDAs as a 'licensing of sin or interference with the providential punishment of vice' (Logan, 1871, p. 220).

This shortcoming had apparently already been noted in Dublin's Lock Hospital, about half a century earlier. The presence of the laundry and the compositional changes to the board of governors suggests a system of moral management had been introduced. At other non-medical institutions, such as the work-house, the prison or the Magdalen Asylum, the principal objectives of a reformation in character and the production of virtue were underpinned by a faith in the redemptive properties of work. Indeed, in the overtly religious Magdalen Asylum, inmates' penitence was measured not only in the chapel, but also in the laundry, where washing and ironing fabric were considered key virtues in the path towards rehabilitation (Figure 83).

The Lock Hospital's shift from a purely medical institution to one which also embodied a redemptive function, reflects and indeed anticipates, the

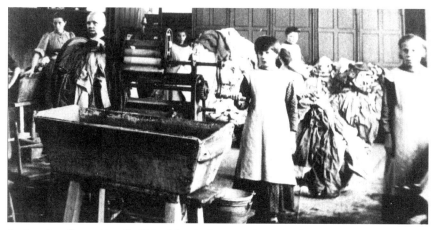

83 Interior of an unidentified Magdalen Asylum in Ireland. (Early twentieth-century image.)

contested perception of prostitution throughout the nineteenth century as it oscillated between one theory, which posited the practice as a medical problem and another, which saw it as a moral and ethical issue (Walkowitz, 1980). In fact, these two schools of thought were not mutually exclusive, but rather tended to influence each other: morality was often inflected with scientific or quasi-scientific data, which in turn, was already coloured by class and gender prejudices. As shall be shown below, both camps often relied on the production of a stream of seemingly objective statistics to justify their respective positions and often investigations into the same phenomena would produce two mutually contradictory proofs. All this contributed to the unique and ambiguous treatment of prostitutes within the medical hospital. While a strict patient discipline was often attempted in most other medical institutions, no other in nineteenth-century Dublin contained a patients' work-place. And, from the 1820s to its ultimate closure in 1952, the Westmoreland Lock occupied an imprecise position somewhere between a reformatory and a hospital, shifting occasionally to accommodate changes in the moral or scientific climates. It is tempting to suggest this ambiguity was also embodied

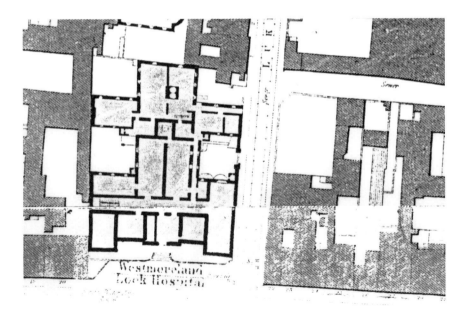

84 Westmoreland Lock Hospital Plan.
(Ordnance Survey 'five-foot' plan, Sheets 15 and 22; 1847.)

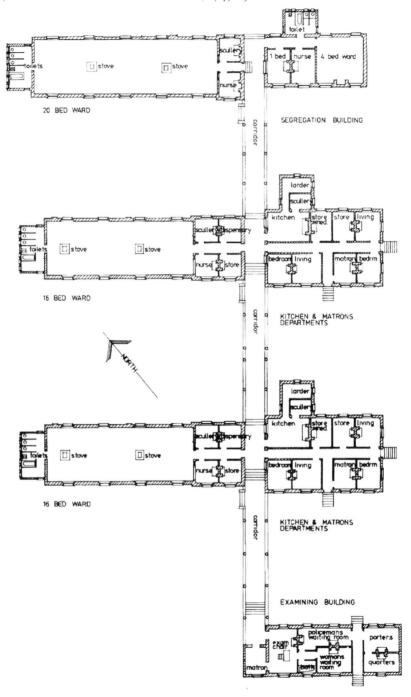

85 The Government Lock Hospital at Kildare, built under the Contagious Diseases Acts, 1869 and closed after their suspension in 1883 (Finnegan, 2001).

in the building itself whose plan, by 1847, seems confused and fragmented and displays little of the rigour of Richard Johnston's (or, to a lesser extent Francis's), interventions (Figure 84). Indeed, one can compare it with the ordered plan of the Kildare Lock Hospital, a pavilion scheme, which opened in a green field site adjacent to the army barracks on the Curragh in 1869 and was constructed under scrupulous medical and military supervision as one of the measures introduced by the CDAs (Finnegan, 2001, pp 114–97) (Figure 85).

Located in the city – hemmed in by streets and other obstacles and further constrained by its relationship with an existing building as well as the fluctuating attitudes towards prostitution – the form of the Westmoreland Lock Hospital was always subject to certain compromises. Ironically, by 1889, even the Hospital for Incurables in Donnybrook had been transformed into a modern pavilion plan. Unburdened by the immoral connotations of prostitution, the patients there had been more successfully subsumed into medicalized objects. And, as the definition of incurable converged with its modern meaning, the hospital assumed more and more the function of the modern hospice, (or, curiously, the *ancien régime* hospital), offering care and succour, often in quite medically progressive ways, to those dying from tuberculosis, cancer or a variety of other terminal illnesses (Burke, 1993, p. 133).

The uproar of the CDAs and their immediate aftermath not only consolidated the association between the prostitute's body and venereal disease, it also gave prostitution a symbolic centrality in the nineteenth-century popular imagination (Walkowitz, 1992, p. 20). Of the manifold books and pamphlets published throughout the century, William Logan's text, *The Great Social Evil* perhaps comes closest to conveying (while also contributing to) the hysteria surrounding the practice. Its title evokes age-old associations of sin and places the prostitute in the vacated position of the leper or madman, as society's principal pariah, a figure of fear, loathing or sympathy. The changes at the Westmoreland Lock Hospital in 1820 seem to foreshadow this development: as the male venereal patients were absorbed into the heterogeneous and more general hospitals of Steeven's and the Richmond Surgical, their female counterparts became the sole inheritors of the specialized and pejorative meanings of the Lock Hospital – associations which were to endure and indeed intensify, until after the building closed in the twentieth century. In James Joyce's *Ulysses*, published in 1922, for instance, a female character of apparently easy virtue is evocatively described as, 'Mary Shortall that was in the Lock with the Pox' (Joyce, 1922).

Visibility and order: other institutions by Francis Johnston

The chain of events which helped to bring about the transformations in the Lock Hospital around the turn of the century – the 1798 rebellion, the Act of Union, the war with France and the subsequent militarization of society – simultaneously influenced the creation or alteration of other spaces and buildings in Dublin. The acceleration of institutional building which the city experienced at this time, has been perceived as part of an attempt to imbue the urban population with a new spirit of obedience. This notion is lent further credence by the revival of the city's forgotten motto *Obientia Civium Urbis Felicitus* (Obedient Citizens Make a Happy City) which was emblematically inscribed into the main gate of one of these institutions, the Richmond House of Correction (Richmond or City Bridewell) on the South Circular Road, on its completion in 1813 (Campbell, 1998, p. 36).

To help achieve this new civil contract of acquiescence, the latest breed of disciplinary institutions were designed with perhaps the most rigorous embodiment of scientific principles witnessed to date in the city. Unencumbered by existing buildings or constraining urban sites, Francis Johnston as Architect of the Board of Public Works, was able to improve on his earlier interventions at both the Foundling and Lock Hospitals and, at the same time, indulge his personal passion for mechanistic devices (Betjemin, 1951), to approach the creation – in the Richmond Penitentiary, the Richmond Lunatic Asylum and the Richmond House of Correction – of what Foucault has termed the 'complete and austere institution'. These were buildings which were conceived as types of apparatus, ones whose very layout and form could efficiently administer to 'all aspects of the individual, his physical training, his aptitude to work, his everyday conduct, his moral attitude, his state of mind' (Foucault, 1977, p. 235; Figure 86). Here, in a parallel process to the evolution of the clinical hospital, the power of the gaze has been inverted to become the generator of interior space and an integral part in a mechanism of control. Foucault also asserted, however, that the scientifically determined institution of the nineteenth century was, in fact, merely the latest incarnation in a long history of deployment of asymmetrical and irrational power over marginal bodies. In Dublin, therefore, the regime of surveillance underpinning Francis Johnston's institutions can perhaps be conceptualized as a modern inflection in a recurring theme of visibility which claimed amongst its antecedents, the brutal and bloody deterring spectacle of old Newgate or the dark and sinister disciplinary theatre of the new Newgate.

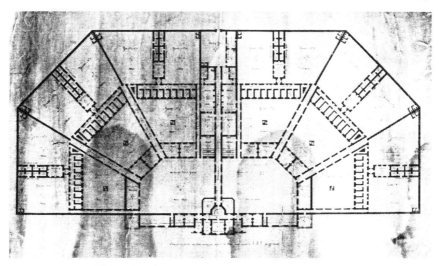

86 Ground floor plan of the Richmond Penitentiary. (Francis Johnston, 1812.)

Moreover, while the main thrust of this disciplinary surveillance was focused on the inmates, the presence of these institutions, as immense hulks moored to the fringes of the city, like the abandoned medieval *leprosia* Foucault cites, simultaneously cast an external symbolic shadow across the rest of the population. Accordingly, traces of the theatricality of Newgate Gaol remained on their public fronts, especially around their entrances, where there was often a stark eruption of architectural elements (or aptly chosen text), which, while relieving the relentless utilitarian façade cannot realistically be called ornamentation. Instead, this architecture of ponderous pediments and heavy rustication exhibited, most notably at the Richmond House of Correction's 'Cease to do Evil Gate' (Figure 87), a reminder to the citizen, not only of the dangers of disobedience, but also of the implacable power and identity of those charged with punishing it. Indeed, as well as having their origins in the brutal superstitions of the past, the dispassionate and scientific pretensions of Johnston's institutions are further refuted by their position within a specific cultural and political climate.

Although it has been acknowledged that the rise of an urbanized industrial society produced a social order whose very complexity forced the adoption of some sort of institutional response (Scull, 1979, p. 14), the proliferation of institutions in Dublin was also irrevocably and inextricably bound up in the 'complex machinations of post-Union politics' (Campbell, 1998, p. 38). Established directly by the government, at a time of war with France and uncertain loyalties, these buildings were more than symbols of civic authority, but rather the potent visual signifiers of direct British control and authority in

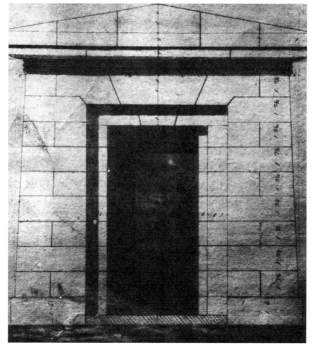

87 'Cease to Do Evil Gate', Richmond House of Correction.
(Francis Johnston, 1811, Irish Architectural Archive.)

Ireland. Perhaps unsurprisingly then, their supposedly rational and mechanistic organisation began to break down almost immediately under the weight of unscientific and partisan practices.

This is perhaps best exemplified in the fate of the Richmond Penitentiary whose precisely calibrated spaces began, soon after its opening, to be overwhelmed by cruder and more pressing demands (Campbell, 1998, p. 62). Firstly, it was closed temporarily amidst allegations that proselytizing and torture were being applied to its Catholic inmates. When it reopened in 1832, the building's internal organization had been significantly changed partly in response to the shifting identity of its prospective inmates and their disorders. In 1832, it became a cholera hospital coping with the victims of the epidemic which swept the city that year. By 1837, however, it had become (and would remain for the next sixty years) the Richmond Female Penitentiary. It was one of many buildings, large and small, which emerged in Dublin over the course of the century in an attempt to solve – through the highly ordered and visible world of the institution – the growing problem of specifically female pathologies and their spatial manifestation in the city.

The creation of Monto

The profligate side effects of militarization in a rapidly growing city, combined with a lack of female employment opportunities due to Dublin's industrial under-development and intensified, perhaps, by the pre-1820 Lock Hospital's implicit acceptance of prostitution and sexual licentiousness, had all contributed to the development of a trade in flesh in the city which by 1820 was burgeoning. Indeed, by the end of the century, it had earned Dublin a notoriety which even found its way into the pages of the tenth edition of the *Encyclopaedia Britannica* (published in 1903), which stated that, in terms of prostitution:

> Dublin furnishes an exception to the usual practice in the United Kingdom. In that city police permit open 'houses' confined to one area, but carried on more publicly than even in the south of Europe or Algeria.

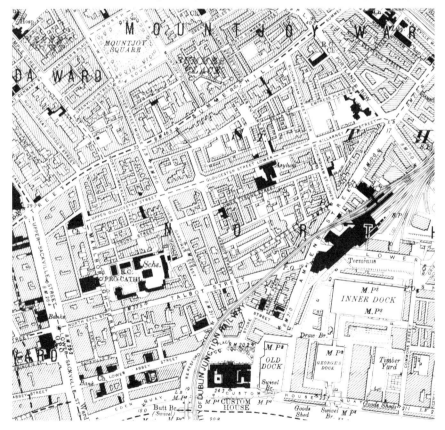

88 Plan showing location of Monto. Sackville Street is on the extreme left and Amiens Street on the right. (Ordnance Survey 1:10, 560 plan, Sheet 18; 1912.)

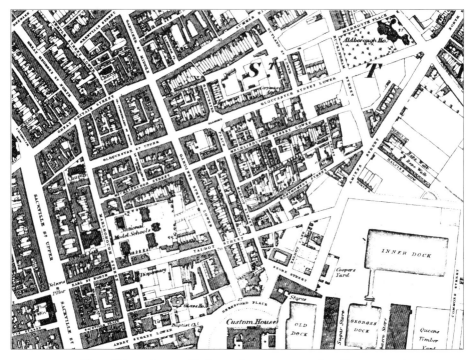

89 Plan of Monto in 1837. (Ordnance Survey 1:10, 560 plan, Sheet 18; 1837.)

The area, known colloquially as Monto (or, alternatively 'the Kips', 'the Digs' or Macktown after Mrs Mack, one of its more infamous denizens) was located just a few hundred yards to the east of Sackville Street. In the mid-nineteenth century, it formed a wedge shaped block of city space bounded: to the east by Mabbot Street; to the west by Buckingham Street; to the north by Mecklenburgh Street; and to the south by Montogomery Street from which it derived its most popular name (Figures 88 and 89).

The area's transformation into its privileged position as the British Isles' only sanctioned zone of iniquity occurred incrementally. Indeed, zones like it had previously flourished, not only in other cities throughout the United Kingdom, but also elsewhere in Dublin. Earlier in the nineteenth century, for example, St Stephen's Green had already achieved a degree of ill-fame as a locus for streetwalking as had Grafton Street, while the nearby French Street had enjoyed a fleeting reputation as a site of brothels, similar to the area surrounding the Royal Barracks (especially Barrack Street) in the city's westward reaches. Towards the end of the century, however, the more visible aspects of prostitution had more or less been cleared from central areas to become almost exclusively concentrated in Monto, albeit with a small scattering of outposts in non-central areas such as the canals and Barrack Street. This coincided with a fall in the arrests of prostitutes in Dublin in the latter stages of the nineteenth century, from a total of 3,255 in 1870 to a total of 431 by 1900 (Dublin Metropolitan Police Statistics, 1838–1900, quoted in Luddy, 1990, p. 57).

This decline has been attributed, at least in part, to two factors: the establishment in Dublin of the White Cross Vigilance Association in 1885 and, the introduction in the same year, of the Criminal Law Amendment Act (Luddy, 1990, p. 57). Both these phenomena reflected a significant shift towards the more absolute moral attitude that the practice of prostitution should be suppressed completely. The White Cross Vigilance Association, like the Association for the Discountenancing of Vice of the previous century, has been described as a 'social-purity' movement, one which was dedicated to the elimination of vicious habits and the general improvement of morality (Walkowitz, 1980, p. 251). Meanwhile, the Criminal Law Amendment Act – designed to replace the Contagious Diseases Acts (suspended in 1884 and repealed completely in 1886) – abnegated its predecessor's tacit toleration of prostitution and instead introduced strict measures to make the operation of brothels illegal and penalize landlords who rented rooms to known prostitutes.

During the last decade of the nineteenth century, the medical conception of prostitution began to be increasingly affected by moral issues. Ironically, this came in the wake of a renewed medical appreciation of venereal disease and the slowly dawning realization that the medically prescribed measures of regulation and treatment, effected through the Contagious Diseases Acts, were not actually able to cure gonorrhoea or syphilis after all. Ultimately, the Acts became perceived as 'institutional incarnations of a flawed and discredited pathology' and medical emphasis shifted more and more to address lifestyle and induce changes in sexual behaviour and social habits, a tendency which endured until the First World War (Walkowitz, 1980, p. 254). The new-found consensus between medical and moral ideologies signalled the death knell for the semi-officially tolerated red-light districts located throughout the British Isles as, between 1890 and 1914, under the aegis of local purity groups and enforced by local authorities, a programme of the systematic repression of brothels unfolded. It is difficult to explain exactly how Monto managed to elude this dragnet. However, in the Criminal Law Amendment Act itself, the authorities charged with implementing the piece of legislation in Dublin appear to be different from those in other British and Irish cities, a circumstance which may offer some clues to the law's apparent lack of enforcement in the Irish metropolis.

In fact, despite the decline in arrests in the last decade of the nineteenth century, apocryphal evidence hints at an actual increase in the activities of the prostitutes in Dublin, if not in their actual number. This occurred especially during the Boer War (1899–1901) as the following ode published in the *Irish Society* magazine suggests. Written on the triumphant return of an Irish regiment, the first letter of every line reveals the less than heroic consequence of the influx of ex-combatants into the city.

> The gallant Irish yeomanry
> Home the war has come
> Each victory gained o'er foeman,
> Why should our bards be dumb?
>
> How shall we sing their praises,
> Or glory in their deeds,
> Renowned their worth amazes,
> Empires their prowess needs.
>
> So to Old Ireland's hearts and homes,
> We welcome now our own braves boys
> In cot and hall; 'neath lordly domes
> Love's heroes share once more our joys.
>
> Love in the Lord of all just now,
> Be he the husband, lover, son,
> Each dauntless soul recalls the vow
> By which not fame, but love was won.
>
> United now in fond embrace
> Salute with joys each well-loved face.
> Yeomen, in women's heart you hold the place
> (*Irish Society,* quoted in Fagan, 2000, p. 20)

While the exact reasons for Monto's location on the north side of Dublin to the east of Sackville Street remain unclear, a number of contributing factors can be discerned. Many of these involve the military. As has been shown, the billeting of part of a notoriously profligate army in the temporarily converted Rotunda during the 1798 rebellion, attracted fresh waves of lower-class prostitutes and camp-followers to an area already imbued with dubious connotations. This in turn presumably acted as a magnet for the thousands of lusty troops drafted in the wake of Robert Emmet's uprising and the French Wars. Monto's position as the city's principal zone of prostitution, however, only really began to be consolidated after the Crimean War had necessitated the conversion of the nearby Aldborough House into a barracks and the central supply station for the British troops in Ireland (Fagan, 2000, p. 10). In 1871, the reformer William Logan's description of a visit to Dublin confirms a particular geographic relationship between prostitution and the army: 'In a back street in a neighbourhood of the Barracks there were, it was said, some 200 of these wretched girls' (Logan, 1871, p. 51). Other, more folkloric accounts of Monto, describe innovative methods of soliciting potential military clients, including the sending of 'calling-cards' to new regiments stationed in the city and the enticing appearance of glamorously attired *demi-mondaines*, at the events in the Dublin social calendar frequented by army officers, such as the Dublin Horse Show or the Fairyhouse or Punchestown Races.

Monto's descent into notoriety took place against a commensurate slide of the entire north side of the city into a vast zone characterized mainly by poverty and deprivation. One of the roots of this transformation lay in the flight of the aristocracy and gentry after the Act of Union as the closure of parliament had denied them their principal reason for remaining. As Prunty (1998) suggests, the nearby presence of such anti-social institutions such as the barracks, the markets, asylums, the fever hospital and the House of Industry may have kept the area on a downward trajectory until it had become what has since been described as a 'classic slum'. The exodus of the rich to the southern and northern suburbs and beyond, left behind a vacated landscape of townhouses which, slowly at first, then with added momentum, began to be colonised by the poor. This process began in the hinterland, where the 'stable-lanes and associated mews buildings which were built to serve the fine front-street houses succumbed easily to low-status residential use'. Soon, however, the townhouses themselves began to be sub-divided into multi-occupancy dwellings. Significant discrepancies between the names and addresses contained in the relief rolls of local charities and those contained in official statistical sources such as the *General Valuation of Ireland* (Griffith's Valuation of 1854) or commercial directories such as Thom's or Shaw's, illustrate what has been described as the 'invisibility of the very poorest' among the landscape of sublets and spatial subdivisions (Prunty, 1998, pp 274–335). The sudden densification in population and the informal altering of buildings by their new occupants to create new routes and spaces, effectively transformed large chunks of the north-side into what appeared to be a vast and disorderly maze hewn in the fabric of the formerly ordered Georgian urban plan. By 1900, only a few zones – such as the commercially orientated Sackville Street or the still fairly affluent Rutland and Mountjoy Squares – had completely escaped the onslaught of being transformed wholesale into tenements.

Statisticians, morality and public space

The relative invisibility of the poor and indeed, the beguiling qualities of their neighbourhoods had been a consistent source of interest to certain sections of the middle classes since the end of the eighteenth century. Indeed, many attempts had been carried out by medical doctors, clergymen, sanitary officers, journalists, philanthropists and others, to inquire into, map, and ultimately reveal to the bourgeois world, the conditions of the poor in the city. Despite the obvious differences in the occupations and specializations of those who carried out the surveys, certain similarities and consistencies have been noted in their descriptions. These, more often than not, introduced the topics as if writing about a foreign land and requested that the reader's belief be suspended as they described the characteristics and peculiarities of the native 'denizens' (Prunty, 1998, p. 18).

The significance of these investigations was periodically reiterated in times of crisis, when the horrors of the slums threatened to escape their boundaries and spill into the wealthier areas of the city. For example, Dublin's first such survey *An Essay on the Population of Dublin*, compiled in 1798 by James Whitelaw, was written not only in the aftermath of a fever epidemic but also in the period of upheaval following the 1798 rebellion. Both conditions perhaps contributed equally to the necessity of increased knowledge of and surveillance into poor areas as neither armed uprising nor infectious fever was a particular respecter of class or social boundaries.

The plethora of surveys and inquiries into the poor, spanning the nineteenth and early twentieth centuries took place against the backdrop of what has been called the statistical revolution. Described in 1814 as 'the knowledge of the present state of a country with a view to its future development' (Mason, 1814, pp vi–viii), the science of statistics was predicated on the belief that through endless and meticulous observation, measurement and recording, the true nature of phenomena could be revealed and thus future trends and developments successfully divined. In technique and theory, therefore, it had similarities to medicine and its triumvirate of examination, diagnosis and prognosis. Indeed, the actual origins of statistical science has been traced to the works of the seventeenth-century physician and author of the *Down Survey*, William Petty, and especially his *Natural and Political Observations on the Bills of Mortality*, (1662), which is often regarded as the prototypical statistical text. In nineteenth-century Dublin, the early surveys and statistical publications, following Whitelaw's *Essay*, tended to be mainly medically-inspired investigations into the relationship between contagious diseases and the environment of the poor. While this type of investigation perhaps reached its zenith in the wake of the Asian Cholera epidemic of 1832–3, the presence of medical officers continued to dominate statistical science in the city as it developed throughout the century. The new era in social investigation ushered in by the Census of Ireland (1841/1851), for example, was instigated and organised by William Wilde, surgeon and author of many texts, including the biographical note on Bartholomew Mosse referred to in chapter 1 above. It has been suggested, however, that from the very beginning, the scientific prerequisites of statistical enquiry – objective and detached observation and recording – were not only inevitably compromised by class and gender bias, but were also subject to deliberate manipulation. Indeed, the original name of 'political arithmetic' seems to suggest more candidly both the uses and limitations of 'statistical science' (Cullen, 1975, p. 5).

Elsewhere in nineteenth-century Europe, investigations into the social phenomena of the unseen city were becoming more specialised. Perhaps unsurprisingly, the figure of the female prostitute and the spaces she inhabited became the focus of a particularly intense level of scrutiny and examination. Described as the Isaac Newton of harlotry, the French physician, A.J.B. Parent-Duchâtelet's study of Parisian prostitutes, *De la Prostitution dans la Ville de Paris* (1836) represented the first and perhaps most scientifically rigorous example in what subsequently developed into a veritable genre of investigative works into the practice. Like any good statistician Parent Duchâtelet attempted to provide as comprehensive a description as possible of the prostitute, her profession and the locations she appropriated in the city, by accumulating and compiling a vast and dazzling array of information, data and maps to address the phenomenon at all scales, from the density of prostitution at an urban level in the *arrondissements* of Paris, to more intimate information about prostitutes' health and the condition of their bodies.

Other subsequent texts ranged from William Acton's medically predicated *Prostitution: Considered in its Moral, Social and Sanitary Aspects* (1870) to more morally minded and evangelical texts such as William Logan's *The Great Social Evil* (1871) mentioned above. Henry Mayhew's magnum opus *London Labour and the London Poor* (1862) also contained a chapter, written by his curiously named assistant Bracebridge Hemyng, dedicated to prostitutes whom he listed under the section entitled 'those who will not work' in the exalted company of 'swindlers, thieves and beggars'. Indeed, texts like these, despite their claims of objectivity, tended to lack the obsessive rigour of Parent-Duchâtelet and it has been suggested that some of the Frenchman's findings were subsequently used as a 'statistical template' on to which subjective personal convictions and agendas were grafted (Walkowitz, 1980, p. 37). As has been shown, studies on prostitution in the nineteenth century did not tend to produce dispassionate discussion but rather invoked deeply held prejudices and belief structures as well as, perhaps, other hidden agendas (see Boyd, 2002, pp 219–24). These in fact often extended beyond the realm of the prostitute into considerations not only of the proper place for women in the city but also into the nature of urban space itself.

It has been suggested that the contradictions and ambiguities presented by the burgeoning industrial city provoked a new middle-class appreciation of the family and domesticity as a bulwark of order in an increasingly anarchic environment (Sennett, 1977). The abrupt division between private and public space which emerged in the nineteenth century was, moreover, simultaneously divided into discrete male and female zones (Wilson, 1991). For the majority of middle-class women, the uncontrolled public realm of the city was increasingly forbidden (unless accompanied by a male chaperon) and they became confined more and more to the intimate predictabilities of the bourgeois home. However, as hinted above, much to the horror of many reformers and social commentators, the domestic, social and sexual restrictions placed on the bourgeois female tended to be largely absent from working-class life. Hemyng, for example, stated, with some apparent distaste, that 'to be unchaste amongst the lower classes is not always a subject of reproach'. Extra marital liaisons, however, were dependent on the existence of extra-domestic communal or public spaces, or, as Hemyng put it: 'low lodging houses', 'penny gaffs or 'low cheap places of amusement where so much evil is sown' (Hemyng in Mayhew, 1862, p. 221). Accordingly, while the views of the Revd William Bevan of Liverpool, who testified to the 'necessity of clearing the streets of prostitutes especially after ten o'clock at night, and entirely on market days' (quoted in

Logan, 1871, pp 179–81) were common, other measures posited by reformers were directed at a more comprehensive control of public, semi-public and communal realms. These included: surveillance of the streets, the regulation of lodging houses, the closure or regulation of 'houses of bad character' (which included coffee-shops) the closure of public parks at dusk, and a widespread suppression of places of amusement and 'low entertainment' (Logan, 1871, p. 124 and Mayhew, 1862, p. 246).

The denigration of public space is perhaps most potently inferred by the contemporary description of prostitutes as 'public women', 'disorderly women' or 'streetwalkers'. Each alludes to a breach in the established spatial order which simultaneously attracts a variety of strong emotional responses: fear, scorn, sympathy or excitement. The figure of the prostitute was the most flagrant disobeyer of the spatial, sexual and moral mores of the middle classes. So much so, she was often considered an actual threat to social order. Parent Duchâtelet, for example, returns again and again in his treatise to the disorder that prostitutes caused, a disorder which he linked directly to the French Revolution. Mayhew agreed, suggesting that the *Society for Suppression of Vice* was established to deal with the demoralizing effects that inflicted the whole of Europe in the wake of the same event. Meanwhile, according to Victor Hugo, two of the first individuals to mount the barricades and become martyred for the cause of revolution in the Paris uprising of 1848, were prostitutes. Indeed, it has been suggested that, 'to the nineteenth-century bourgeoisie the "red whore" was one of the most frightening spectres of urban life' (Wilson, 1991, p. 48). That such a dangerous figure might exist unseen at the heart of society, therefore, was a source of special anxiety. Mayhew, Logan, Acton and other writers all devote lengthy sections of their texts to probe the problems of what they called 'clandestine prostitution'. In fact, both Logan and Mayhew denote the unfettered sexual activities of 'amateurs'; 'maid servants, female operatives, milliners, dress-makers, slop-women, or those who do work for cheap tailors', etc. as 'the most serious side of "prostitution"' (Mayhew, 1862, p. 217 and Logan, 1871, p. 255). Here, the dangers of uncontrolled public space were at their most potent, allowing groups of young women to slip in and out of sexual relationships on a casual and part-time basis, more or less invisibly. Moreover, to reformers' ultimate chagrin, these activities often arose out of active desire rather than passive economic necessity and accordingly, they attracted unreserved condemnation: 'A thousand and one causes may lead to a woman's becoming a professional prostitute, but if a woman goes wrong without any cogent reason for so doing, there must be something wrong in her composition, and inherently bad in her nature …' (Logan, 1871, p 255).

The anxiety connected to the ambiguous identity of the amateur prostitute, however, was paralleled by a concern to root out, define and make visible the concealed presence of prostitution within heterogeneous areas of the city. By closely studying streets and building fabric, Logan, in particular, considered himself able to discern the subtle differences which indicated the presence of a brothel – window blinds drawn at odd hours, for example, or lights blazing late at night in a house when all others in the street were extinguished. His spirit of investigation, however, also took him into more disorientating, labyrinthine environments.

> I got down on my hands and knees and moved along very slowly and cautiously till I reached the other end of the plank, when I felt something like a stair, and finding myself right in my conjectures started to ascend. I fancied that the people above had heard my movements, for the sound of voices as of persons talking in a sort of whisper still reached me. Arrived at the top of the stair I knocked at what turned out to be the door, which was opened, and I observed at a glance that the house was a third-class brothel, in which I found several young men and young women.
>
> (Logan, 1871, p. 31)

Monto: labyrinth of vice?

Despite mentions of Dublin in reformers' text about prostitution or mentions of prostitution in similar texts about Dublin, neither the practice nor its concentration in Monto was written about in detail until the early twentieth century. Even then, its first and most famous committal to paper was not through the pen of a reformer but by James Joyce, reflecting the attraction of such areas, not only to social reformers, but also to that other breed of middle-class adventurer: the stroller or flâneur. Joyce visited the area twice in his works; stumbling across it for the first time in *A Portrait of the Artist as a Young Man* (1916) then later using it as the setting for the 'Nighttown' or 'Circe' chapter in *Ulysses* (1922).

> The Mabbot street entrance to Nighttown, before which stretches an uncobbled tramsiding set with skeleton tracks, red and green will-o'-the-wisps and danger signals. Rows of flimsy houses with gaping doors. Rare lamps with rainbow fans. Round Rabaiotti's halted ice gondola stunted men and women squabble. They grab wafers between which are wedged lumps of coal and copper snow. Sucking they scatter slowly.

Children. The swancomb of the gondola, highreared, forges through the murk, white and blue under a lighthouse. Whistles call and answer.
(Joyce, 1992, pp 562–3)

Joyce's nightmarish and surrealist depiction in *Ulysses* plays upon aspects of Monto which were the source not only of nineteenth-century reformist fears and anxieties but also of the excitement of transgression experienced by the more louche middle-class visitor. He consolidated Monto's character as an 'Other' place by exaggerating already distorted time and gender relationships – Monto is not only 'Nighttown', in contradistinction to the day, but it is also a public space in the city infused with feminine, as opposed to masculine, characteristics. This remains pejorative. The decision to place his version of Homer's Circe, the emasculating and animal-creating witch within Monto, re-emphasises the popular bourgeois perception, that such places of ill-repute were injurious to the nation's manhood. Perhaps unsurprisingly, Joyce's fantastic landscape of crones, transvestites, talking animals and other social and physical misfits, which seems to play upon the wilder flights of fancy of the nineteenth-century *exposé*, found a subsequent echo in the writings of a reformer. Religious zealot, founder member of the, quasi-military, Catholic organization the Legion of Mary and ultimate nemesis of Monto, Frank Duff's memoirs of his activities in the area in the 1920s are strewn with evocations of weirdness and unnaturalness. In the following excerpt, for example, illicit drinking in a shebeen is recast as a 'witches' Sabbath'.

There ensued what was like a religious rite – so solemnly was it carried out. They ranged themselves round in a circle then silence reigned. The carrier of the methylated spirit bottle stood inside that circle … There they were, rigid except for trembling hands, their eyes staring out of their heads, all riveted on the methylated spirit and following its circulatory progression. It was just as if the Blessed Sacrament were being carried round a room full of good people; every eye would be fixed on the blessed sacrament. The craving of their souls for the drink was in their faces. As each one's turn came, the glasses were passed to her and convulsively clutched as if life itself depended on the elixir which was at that moment gurgling out of the big black bottle into the little glass. This proceeding was repeated until all had got their share. Then a regular witches' dance started … Round and round until the little breath they had gave out.
(Duff, June 1940, p. 6)

Suspension of conventional social/spatial boundaries in Monto meant a rare moment of intersection between the social classes. It was one of the few places within the poorer districts where the upper-class gentlemen would congregate and mix openly with men and women from so-called inferior backgrounds. At the moment of its ultimate suppression, for instance, a member of parliament was among those arrested. Moreover, prostitutes themselves could occasionally be of an upper-class pedigree, brought low by some chance or misdemeanour. The area also contained a further gender inversion. Unlike the city which was controlled by city fathers, according to Duff, Monto was governed by a powerful matriarchy of madams who controlled both prostitutes and clients (Duff, September 1940, p. 5). These social distortions, furthermore, seemed to be embodied and signified in the transformations exercised upon the built fabric of the area as it descended into poverty. In Monto, in common with much of the north-inner city, the alleyways and service lanes, designed as subservient spaces to the main streets of the Georgian townscape, assumed an equal functional importance, despite obvious differences in width and architectural treatment (Figure 90).

Ground floor hallways, for example, often became shortcuts between parallel streets, opening up a myriad of alternative route-ways so that the edges of the private zone did not begin at the front door of the house but, rather,

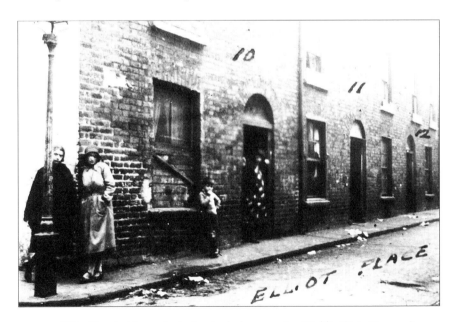

90 Elliot Place in Monto, in decline in the late twenties. (Dublin Civic Museum.)

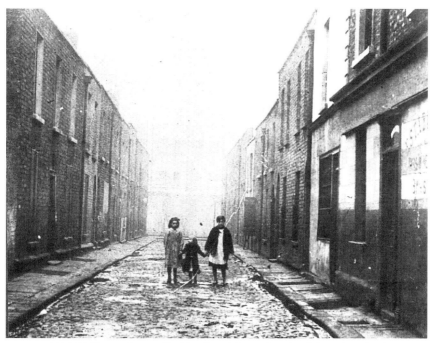

91 Faithful Place in Monto (Dublin Civic Museum). Behind these dour façades, according to Duff, lay sumptuous premises.

whole blocks of tenements became almost infinitely penetrable. Joyce's description of 'flimsy houses with gaping doors' effectively sexualizes these distortions, implying that the availability of intercourse was reflected within the very built fabric as physical thresholds were diminished to the same degree as social ones. Such transformations were impossible to read from maps because they were created unofficially and without formal planning: an incremental appropriation of space, almost it seems, in mockery of the precisely ordered spaces of the Georgian city. The organic nature of this dense occupancy begins to explain why Monto is described again and again by Joyce in animalistic terms, as lairs, warrens, nests etc., 'figures wander, lurk, peer from warrens' (Joyce, 1992, p. 562). The application of the animal metaphor, however, is not unique. Again Joyce, perhaps unconsciously, has appropriated the emotive language of the nineteenth-century reformer: 'Shadwell, Spitalfields, and contiguous districts are infested with nests of brothels …' (Mayhew, 1862, p. 230).

At the centre of such descriptions is an apparent anxiety concerning invisibility and the diminishment of the visual sense: 'warrens' and 'lairs' imply non-rectilinear space, a space of impaired vision where other sensual qualities are heightened. Indeed, one of the reformer's basic premises was that he entered the dark areas of the city in order to bring them to the light of the public gaze and consciousness. Duff suggests that artifice and deceit were central to the functioning of Monto. The illicit nature of many of its activities meant that the area tended to remain hidden from the rest of the city. Monto was located in a unfashionable area, safely removed from the everyday life of those with delicate sensibilities. Brothels and illegal drinking dens did not announce their presence on to the public realm but rather existed behind dowdy masks. According to Duff, ordinary-looking doors in shabby streets sometimes opened into magnificent and opulent rooms – 'a whirlwind of life … a horrible glamour' – which often imitated the decorative trends of the Parisian brothels (Duff, Christmas 1939, p. 4; Figure 91).

In comparison with the 'honest poverty' of the surrounding streets, Monto was the locus of a relative wealth manifesting itself in what Duff called a 'spurious glitter' which concealed 'the underlying filth'. His description was extended to some of the women themselves, who, like the brothels located in former bourgeois houses, aped the appearance of respectable upper-class society while being subject to the 'universal defilement of disease'.

> The life of these girls is often imagined to be one of glamour and pleasure. What fine dresses, gay effects, loud laughter, 'a good time', nothing to do but enjoy themselves! But no distorting mirror ever reflected a more crooked image than that!
>
> (Duff, Christmas 1940, p. 10)

The disorientating and labyrinthine spaces experienced by male middle-class reformers in the nineteenth century, however, may have been a product of their own fertile imaginations (Walkowitz, 1980 and Wilson, 1991). While, to outsiders, like Joyce, the libertine stroller or Duff, the outraged reformer, areas like Monto represented a scarcely decipherable network, to those who lived there, it contained a perfectly reasonable and legible logic. Obliged by conditions of poverty and dense occupation to live more communally, working class perceptions of public/private space were perhaps more fluid than their middle-class counterparts. Indeed, it seems that the nineteenth-century bourgeois explorer's amusement or outrage at what they experienced in the poorer areas was based primarily on their own preconceived perceptions of normality. Accordingly, descriptions of areas of vice or, indeed, simply poor areas are full of what now seems to be exaggeration and fantasy. Monto is characteristically represented by its night-time activities despite the fact that for a long time it contained a heterogeneous population and a mundane daytime existence which seldom involved any impropriety (Fagan, 2000). The prostitution profile of Monto itself, may be an exaggeration to serve as an icon of 'Otherness': the practice assumed the same symbolic centrality in representations of Monto, as it did in the late nineteenth-century consciousness.

The presence of three magdalen asylums and female penitentiaries within the precincts of Monto, as well as numerous other institutions scattered throughout the city, reveals perhaps that the spirit of *laissez-aller* indulgence, apparently shown Monto by the British authorities, was not universally shared. Indeed, despite or because of the apparent non-enforcement of the Criminal Law Amendment Act, private and religious social-purity activism – whose mission was to redeem and resurrect the fallen and sinful – flourished in the city in the late-nineteenth and early-twentieth centuries. It has been suggested that the nationwide furore surrounding the Contagious Diseases Acts and the moral backlash which followed them, conspired to shift the practice of prostitution, from mainly informal and temporary forms – entered into and left according to needs and very much an accepted part of working-class society – into a discrete and isolated profession (Walkowitz, 1980). Under intense middle-class scrutiny, it was no longer possible for women to pass freely from one side to the other without definite consequences. Accordingly, the figure of the prostitute became more unambiguously defined as part of a homogeneous and concentrated group of hardened and habitual outcasts.

Monto, to a large extent, shared this experience, shrinking and concentrating its activities in its latter stages, before, under strong consensual pressure from the Legion of Mary and the Dublin Metropolitan Police, finally giving up the ghost in the early 1920s and scattering some of its seed back into the city. By the 1930s, the entire area had been razed, many of the street names changed, two of its streets completely obliterated and its maze-like warren of alleys and routes replaced with orthogonal and highly visible blocks of flats placed within open space and each with a single entrance (Figure 92) – characteristics which were not too dissimilar to the architecture of Francis Johnston's late institutions such as the Richmond House of Correction.

Monto's destruction after the end-point of British rule in Ireland (1921) is fitting. Its existence was irrevocably entwined with the convergence of British and Irish interests surrounding the Act of Union. It was a by-product of the military presence necessary to keep Ireland loyal and in line. The authorities' implicit tolerance of the area and their general reluctance to interfere,

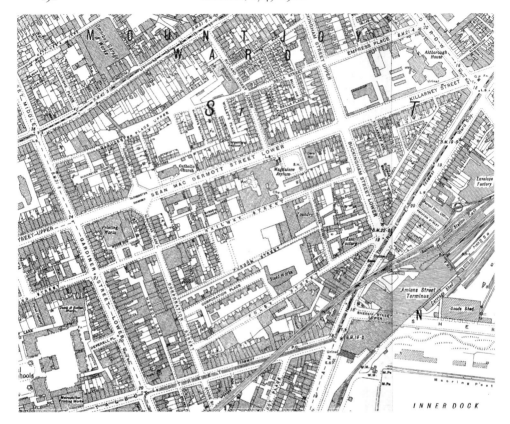

92 Plan of Monto in the 1930s, with missing streets and copious demolitions.
(Ordnance Survey 1:2500 plan, Sheets 18 vii and 18 viii; 1938.)

however, had brought its own problems. Monto was characterized by a general lawlessness which made it difficult for policemen and soldiers to enter unless strictly on unofficial business and ironically, some of its most potent dangers were ultimately reserved for its best and most loyal customers. According to some of the contributors to a recently produced oral history, the area was used as a listening-post by the Irish rebels during the War of Independence (1919–21), when soldiers would inadvertently disclose details about troop movements or counter-espionage to their female escorts, who in turn relayed the information to the insurgent forces. (Fagan, 2000, pp 75–90). The spectre of the revolutionary 'red whore', then, is replaced by a verdant nationalist version who, as well as haunting the nightmares of the bourgeoisie, surreptitiously disrupted the imperial project. But, while her presence in the city was accommodated, it was contingent on her confinement to its hidden backlands. The first Catholic Chief Commissioner of the Dublin Metropolitan Police, Lieutenant Colonel Sir John Foster Ross of Bladensburg's abortive and premature attempt to clean up Monto before independence, had met with cries of indignation centred around the fear that the contents of the suppressed red-light district would spill out to pollute the entire city. This reaction was partly provoked by the sight of streetwalking prostitutes candidly soliciting under the portico of the General Post Office in Sackville Street during the period of the police raids (Duff, Christmas 1939, p. 6 and March 1941, p. 7). Evidently, the presence of such disorderly emissaries from backstage Dublin was deeply unacceptable at such a totem of civic respectability and symbol of empire.

Epilogue

The city as theatre

In 1769, John Bush suggested that if Sackville Street was to be extended to the river, it would perhaps be 'one of the grandest and most beautiful streets in Europe'. In 1818, twenty years after such an extension was made, Warburton, Whitelaw and Walsh – in their description of the urban panorama on offer to any visitor who chose to view the city from Carlisle Bridge – seemed to concur, suggesting that: 'strangers who visit Dublin are especially struck with the beauty of this assemblage of objects … on the south are to be seen, at the termination of Westmoreland Street, the perspective façades on each side of the College and House of Lords; on the east, the front of the Custom-house, which an accidental flexure of the river presents obliquely in a most striking point of view. On the north, the noble perspective of Sackville-street terminated by the Rotunda, and ornamented with the new Post-office and Nelson's Pillar' (1818, p. 1082).

The additions of the pediment and portico of the General Post Office and the antique simplicity of Nelson's Pillar imbued 'the noble perspective' of Sackville Street, more than ever before, with the formal gravitas of columns, pediments, statues and other royal surroundings which Vitruvius had deemed necessary for the creation of the tragic scene (Figure 93). Indeed, when viewed from Carlisle Bridge, even the spire of St Georges Church in Hardwicke Place (designed by Francis Johnston between 1802 and 1813), broke the skyline at a location compositionally reminiscent of the obelisk which appears in Serlio's rendering of the tragic perspective (Figure 94). At the same time as the additions of the General Post Office and Nelson's Pillar were adding to the magnificence of Sackville Street and accentuating its relationship to the tragic scene, they were, however, also altering the meaning of this urban space.

In the first decade of the nineteenth century, Francis Johnston collaborated with William Wilkins on the design of the monument to Lord Nelson. Built to commemorate Nelson's death and victories, the pillar was a stark and monumental edifice: a large fluted shaft in the Doric order, surmounted by a statue of the hero, which dominated the centre of the street. Unlike Wellington, Nelson had no personal connections to Ireland. Rather, his sculptural presence included Dublin (and Ireland) in the celebrations of the

EPILOGUE

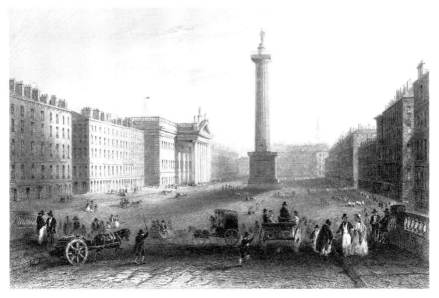

93 View of Sackville Street from Carlisle Bridge. (Bartlett, 1835.)

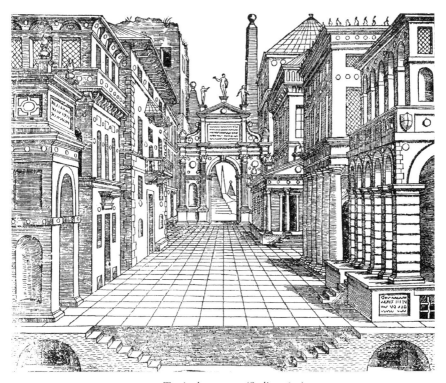

94 Tragic theatre set. (Serlio, 1611.)

triumphs of British military might (Whelan, 2003, pp 44–6). By 1816, the monument's Doric shaft had been joined in the streetscape by the Ionic portico of the General Post Office (GPO), whose foundation stone had been laid on 12 August 1814, amidst great celebrations, by the earl of Whitworth, lord lieutenant, on the former site of one of Sackville Street's rows of terraced houses. An impressive building, its form and decoration were described in detail by Warburton, Whitelaw and Walsh, who as well as commenting on the unusual haste with which it was built, paid special attention to the portico, which '[projected] from the body of the building so as to range with the street' and the pediment, which was 'ornamented with the Royal Arms in high relief' (1818, p. 1005).

It has been suggested that there is a marked similarity in form between the General Post Office and Francis Johnston's designs for his institutional buildings – such as the Richmond House of Correction – which were being executed at about the same time. Both exhibit what Edward McParland has described as the architect's 'penitentiary style'. McParland cites a common treatment of façade which, stripped of ornament, displayed a severe and utilitarian character. In the General Post Office, this was relieved only by the florid gesture of the portico. But even here, in its latter stages, the design was altered from the opulent Corinthian Order to the more severe Ionic (1969, p. 128; Figure 95).

This relationship, however, perhaps extends beyond the merely stylistic. Like Johnston's institutions, it was a centralized British administration which ultimately controlled this new space. This was emphatically registered in the architecture of the building: from the stark utilitarian façade and the presence of the royal coat of arms contained in the tympanum, to the appropriation of Gandon's overhanging portico motif at the former House of Lords – symbol

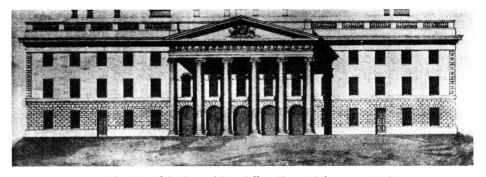

95 Elevation of the General Post Office. (Francis Johnston, *c*.1814.)

of independent Irish governance – and its recasting as part of an instrument of direct British control. If, for Murray Fraser, the architecture of some of the interventions of the Wide Streets Commissioners had represented a tightening of the Gordian knot of British and Irish interests, then it had been, for the most part, a process which was strewn with ambiguities – a sort of imperialism by stealth. The urban form of post-Union Sackville Street – complete with the architecture of the General Post Office and Nelson's Pillar – was less self-conscious in acknowledging its loyalties and indeed, appeared to actively celebrate the demotion of Dublin from a capital to a subaltern city.

There has been then a theatrical consistency throughout all of Sackville Street's manifestations: from the exclusive and discrete suburb, to the principal avenue of a semi-autonomous Protestant Dublin, to a site of State and imperial spectacle. Each represented an attempt to establish a magnificent, spectacular city which celebrated and reflected the identity of a certain class or ideology. In each, however, the architecture and urban space used to prescribe such meanings was subject to subsequent appropriation and subversion – a trend which would endure, with the events of Easter 1916, into the twentieth century (Boyd, 2003).

Backstage Dublin

But while some of the political *detournements* of Sackville/O'Connell Street reflected the application of new ideologies or systems of administration, they were all accompanied by more organic, incremental and enduring appropriations which simply reflected conditions of everyday life in the city. By 1850, for example, the influence of commerce ensured that the uniform façades of the Wide Streets Commissioners' Sackville Street had become disjointed and individualized – as buildings began to be used as sites of advertizing, each competed, with increasingly elaborate decoration and signage, to achieve a visual prominence. This effectively usurped the Commissioners' plan of a unified streetscape punctuated by key civic moments (Figure 96). Perhaps more potently, there was also the persistent re-appearance of marginalized groups, such as the beggars mentioned by Taafe or the prostitutes soliciting under the General Post Office's portico. Their presence provided an explicit reminder of the hidden city of disease, poverty and vice which successive administrations, whatever their associated political ideologies or cultural affiliations, had singularly been unable to control. Each testified to the limitations of the city as a 'harmonious work of art' (Boyer, 1996, p. 78).

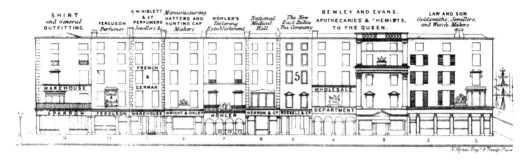

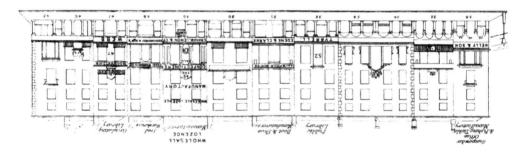

96 Elevation of Sackville Street, 1850. (From Shaw's *Pictorial Dublin Guide and Directory*.)

Walter Benjamin's observation that 'to live is to leave traces' evokes the accumulative nature, not only of the city's inhabitants, but also the city itself (Benjamin, 1939). Consisting of additive layers of material and meaning, the urban process effectively militates against ideal and pure versions of space and instead produces environments of competing narratives and conflicting meanings – of ambiguity, complexity, contradiction and expediency. It has been shown how the attempts of the Anglo-Irish ruling class to impose a singular, concise and self-reflecting narrative on the city created a magnificent landscape punctuated with built superlatives: 'the first', 'the biggest', 'the most grand', 'the most innovatory' etc. The production of this landscape which attempted to defy history and critique by implying, through the remaking of space, that the new order had natural, inevitable and eternal properties, was never fulfilled. Attempts to create a pure architectural embodiment of the identity of the ruling class were compromised not only by having to act within an existing cultural and social matrix, but also by the internal pressures caused by the whims and caprices of the individual members of that class.

The Hospital for Incurables, Cooley's Newgate Gaol, Francis Johnston's carceral institutions, etc., all testify to an attempt to contain, control or reform the agents of disorder, those troublesome elements in the urban mêlée who disrupted the ether of the beautiful city. All failed on their own terms; the Hospital for Incurables degenerated into hopeless squalor as did Newgate Gaol, while Johnston's Enlightenment ideals broke down under the pressure of localised prejudices. Other institutions, however, were more ambiguous. The early years of the Westmoreland Lock Hospital testified to a quasi-official sanctioning of prostitution which was confirmed by the tolerance offered to, and the longevity of, Monto. Similarly, under the cloak of charity and benevolence, agendas of social engineering and experimentation, as well as lust and decadence, informed the history and development of the Lying-in Hospital. Side-by-side with official narratives of munificence, charity and altruism, therefore, emerges a city which also owed its development to more basic but enduring instincts of passion, greed, envy and narcissism.

Benjamin's phrase 'to live is to leave traces', however, does not allude to the relative quality, pervasiveness or visibility of these traces. Throughout this book, inhabiting the sites of magnificence, are the mute historical witnesses who, while contributing to the life of the city and its development, often only have the lines in dusty old ledger books to attest to their existence. These include the peasants and small-farmers cleared from their lands under the onslaught of eighteenth-century agricultural change and whose presence in the city not only swelled its size, but also provoked new theories on population and provided the impetus for new, institutional accommodation. More specifically, there are the mothers and expectant women who experienced the Lying-in Hospital and the prostitutes and 'fallen women' who underwent medical treatment at the Westmoreland Lock Hospital, moral treatment in the Magdalen Asylums or simply walked the streets of Monto. Had they been able to speak, this largely female group, would have undoubtedly shed an entirely different light on the material contained here. For this exploration, however, it was only possible to be constantly aware of how their presence made its mark on the public architecture and urban space of the city. And while much of this may have represented the embodiment of upper class, male attitudes towards the female lower classes as objects of desire, of disorder or productive entities (as we have seen these categories were not mutually exclusive but rather often overlapped and influenced each other), there is also evidence of active female agency: the manipulations of Mrs Leeson in the sexual economy of the time were presumably replicated in other prostitutes including those who brazenly walked the public street, and who provoked the wrath of upright citizens, who in turn introduced measures designed to control their freedom. Even in the disciplinary environment of the Westmoreland Lock Hospital, one can witness, by examining the records, moments of resistance, comfort and perhaps solidarity in the manifold instances of 'irregular conduct' or other misdemeanours between inmates. The relative paucity of their traces, however, not only tends to consign these women to victim-hood, but also underplays their influence in the developing city.

This has been exacerbated by traditional architectural histories whose narrow focus on the planned aspects of building and urban space have perhaps limited our understanding of the city. Non-planned elements, encompassing those unofficial activities which almost inevitably appropriate public space, have tended to remain evasive, elusive and under-discussed. An 'official' description of the Lying-in Hospital and gardens, for example, concentrating only on its much discussed architectural elements or its contribution to the development of midwifery would be a rather sterile and one-dimensional account – lacking the rich complexity of a narrative of medicine, colonialism, consumerism, religion, entertainment and sex, not to mention certain individuals' personal quirks, fancies and insecurities. The lack of hard historical evidence or sworn affidavits from contemporary eye-witnesses means, however, that a deeper appreciation of the Lying-in Hospital, similar institutions or indeed historic urban space, can only be garnered by extending the scope of investigation to encompass a broad sweep of cultural phenomena, allowing new connections to be made, personal histories to be placed into social contexts and apparently arbitrary moments of intersection or coincidence to reveal their true significance.

Contemporary Dublin is immersed, along with many other cities, in a perpetual global competition to attract tourist revenue. One of the many consequences of this is the tendency for the city to attempt to conform to a pre-manufactured image – a city spectacle and conspicuous consumption which apparently seeks to emulate those choreographed depictions proffered in tourist literature. Accordingly, Dublin's city centre has witnessed new methods in controlling public space. These have included the proliferation of surveillance technologies and the closing down of facilities such as public toilets. Allied with the increased privatization of the public realm, this is leading to the creation of a tamed and predictable landscape, shorn of diversity and tolerating only officially prescribed functions. The very elements which have hitherto been omitted from architectural and urban histories of

Dublin but which have, as we have seen, contributed so much to its development, are now being excluded from the city itself. Indeed, in the absence of a readily identifiable hegemonic ruling class – such as the Anglo-Irish or the British Empire – the traces of the marginalized, the dispossessed and the excluded provide the most potent basis for a critique of undemocratic spatial practices, which, perhaps more than ever before, present themselves as natural, ahistorical and inevitable.

APPENDIX 1

Extracts from the Dublin Journal, *5–8 June 1746*

From the Hospital for poor Lying-in Women in Georges-lane, Dublin. This Hospital having hitherto been supported by Collections at Plays and one Musick Meeting and by private Benefactions; the Governors thinks it a Justice due to the Public to give an Account of the Money they have received and how they have applied the same for the Use of the Hospital together with an Account of the Progress and present state of the said Hospital which is as follows: Admitted into the Lying-in Hospital from 25 March 1745 to the 1st July 1746 from the different Parishes the following numbers:

From St Andrew's	24
St Ann's	2
St Audeon's	16
St Bridget's	19
St Catherine's	40
St James's	5
St John's	5
St Luke's	19
St Mark's	5
St Mary's	14
St Michael's	8
St Michan's	10
St Nicholas without	9
St Nicholas within	2
St Paul's	17
St Peter's	12
St Werburgh's	2
Total	209

Amongst these:

Wives of Soldiers and Seamen mostly abroad in His Majesty's Service	41
Poor widows of Soldiers and Seamen killed in His Majesty's Service	14
Wives of Poor Weavers, Combers and Dyers etc.	46
Wives of Poor tradesmen	57
Wives of Poor Servants	24
Widows of Tradesmen, Servants, Labourers etc	8
Wives of poor Men in the Marshalsey	4
From England	6
From Scotland	3
From the Isle of Man	2
Total Admitted	209
Delivered in the Hospital at the same Time	204
Delivered of Boys	114
Delivered of Girls	94
Total born	208

Discharged 191 Women with 105 boys and 85 Girls all very well.
Died one Woman of Fever twelve days after she was safely delivered.
Died 7 Children of Fits
Remain in the Hospital 17 Women, 12 of whom are delivered, and 5 not yet delivered, and 11 children.

To cash received by two Plays and the Oratario of Hester	£330 5s. 6½d.
Do. received by Subscriptions and small private benefactions	£54 7s. 5d.
Total received	£384 12s. 11½d.

Paid towards repairing and fitting up the Hospital and building a Wash-house	£64 4s. 3d.
Paid for necessary furniture, and 16 beds, Bedding etc.	£130 18s. 6d.
Do. for House Expenses for Provisions etc., and Servants Wages	£209 10s. 4½d.
Paid for one year's rent of the Hospital ending 25 March 1746	£30 0s. 0d.
Total expended	£437 13s. 1½d.
Total received	£384 12s. 11½d.
	£53 0s. 0d.
To answer which there are due by tickets and Subscriptions	£104 7s. 8d.

APPENDIX II

Extracts from the Lying-in Hospital Account Book, 1757 (Rotunda Hospital Records)

Account No. 1, Expenses of Beds in the Attick Storie

Grayson, Booth and Co. for sheeting	£77 18s. 9d.
John Newett for checkr. Linnen for Summer Curtains	£57 1s. 0d.
Daniel Dickinson for ditto and Ticken for Mattresses	£46 7s. 5½d.
Alderman Allen for Green Serge for Quilts	£27 17s. 1d.
Terne. Mooney for double Blankets, Kilkenny Blanket, Green Bages and Serge	£75 19s. 1d.
Nath. Trumble for Kitterminster for Winter Curtains	£48 3s. 4d.
Mr. Harford for Hair for the Matresses	£27 13s. 0d.
Cash for flocks for the Quilts	£1 15s. 11½d.
Mrs Moorehead for making Mattresses	£26 12s. 0d.
George Spring's Bill	£15 19s. 10d.
Iron Work at 8/2 for Bed/Fifty-two Beds	£25 6s. 10d.
Wood Work at £3 for ditto	£156 0s. 0d.
Painting Work at 8/1/0 for ditto	£25 2s. 6d.
Linnen for Pillow, Cases, Shift, Caps, Aprons etc	£45 4s. 5½d.
Lace, Tapes, nonesopretty [?], Curtain Rings, and making Sheets, Blankets, Boulsters, pillows and pillow Cases, filling ditto with feathers, the Quilter etc	£28 8s. 2d.
Total	£673 9s. 3d.

Account No. 3, Expenses of Opening the Hospital, the 8 December, 1757.

Confectioners, Cake Makers, Bread, Butter and Cream etc.	£21 10s. 5½d.
Hire and Breaking of China to Mrs White	£4 8s. 8½d.
Carpeting to Mr Dan White	£27 15s. 3d.
Groceries to Mrs Birch	£7 5s. 3d.
Mrs brooks for 1400 tickets	£1 8s. 0d.
Musick and Singers	£14 12s. 3½d.
Labourers, Birch Brooms etc.: cleaning the Streets, Women cleaning the House, Bill Porters, Guards, Elizabeth Knight for her Cloaths etc.	£7 8s. 9½d.
Making the women's cloath and linen to Mrs Smart £8 15s. 6d. and Muningham [?] 5/5	£9 0s. 11d.
Flanells to Mrs Bermingham	£8 3s. 2d.
Ditto and Petty-coats to Mrs Mooney	£15 3s. 0d.
Printing Work to Mr Powell	£1 10s. 0d.
Groceries to James Hamilton	£12 15s. 8d.
Roast Beef, Tongue, Hams, bread and ale	£3 8s. 10d.
2 Dozen Wines and Carriage to Alderman Hamilton	£2 0s. 6d.
Sam Wheatley Engraver for a plate for Tickets	£0 11s. 4½d.
Total	£167 17s. 27½d.

Bibliography

A variety of original sources and types of material were consulted in the production of this book. These range from medical sources such as hospital records, extracts from personal memoirs, newspapers periodicals and other contemporary observations and reports, to urban maps and architectural drawings. The majority of this material is contained in a series of archives and depositories located in the city of Dublin itself.

The principal hospital archives used were the Rotunda Hospital Records, which are contained in the National Archives and the Westmoreland Lock Hospital Records, which are kept in the library of the Royal College of Physicians. As a consequence of the many functions of the Lying-in Hospital such as the Pleasure Gardens etc., the Rotunda Hospital Records contain a diverse range of material including: patient registers, practitioners' notebooks etc., accounts books and details concerning the everyday functioning of the hospital, material to do with entertainment, and work carried out in the gardens, as well as examples of lottery tickets and evidence from other fund-raising schemes. Consulting these records is a convoluted, sometimes rewarding, and sometimes frustrating task. Firstly, because of the sensitivity of some of the later medical records, one must apply in writing to the Master of the Rotunda Hospital to view the collection which, furthermore, can only be accessed at the National Archives on Bishop Street. The records are not adequately catalogued and since they come in large boxes within which are contained bundles of documents, the researcher does not know exactly what they are going to contain. Hence, the sense both of frustration and excitement when one discovers something which, either was not asked for, or was not listed, but turns out to be very important. One example of this was the notebook of D.M.M. (mentioned in chapter 1 above). At other times, however, items which were listed as being in a certain box or bundle were missing. A more detailed catalogue and the further classification of material (some rudimentary work was done in this regard by Edward McParland) would aid the researcher's task considerably and quite possibly reveal other hidden nuggets of material. Finally, the storage of some of this material, in cardboard boxes, envelopes, tied bundles and, in one case, a plastic bag, will ultimately be to its detriment.

What remains of the Westmoreland Lock Hospital Records is a series of bound volumes kept at the Royal College of Physicians Library in Kildare Street. One explanation for the incompleteness of these records which span from 1792 to 1924 is given by the present librarian of the Royal College of Physicians, Robert Mills. According to him, on the closure of the hospital (by then renamed the hospital of St Margaret of Cortona) in the 1950s, the records were in the process of being burned, starting with the most recent, when a passing physician halted the process and donated the remnants to the college. This piece of apocryphal evidence is symptomatic of an apparent sense of shame towards this Dublin institution which perhaps extended itself to the city's historians. Until the publication of this book, no major piece of research had been carried out on the Westmoreland Lock Hospital, perhaps the only major hospital in the city to be so treated (Jones and Malcolm, eds., 1999, p. 11). Perhaps as a consequence of this, there is no catalogue for the hospital's records which include: patient registers, board room minutes (some volumes of which are titled, others are not), chaplains' visiting books, other visiting books, accounts and cashbooks etc. The fragmentary nature of the records is best revealed by the dates covered by the material. The latest patient register, for example, ends in 1875 while the board room minutes contain material from intermittent periods between 1792 until 1909.

A series of drawings for the Westmoreland Lock Hospital by Francis Johnston – along with drawings of many of Johnston's other buildings including his later institutions – are contained in the Murray Collection in the Irish Architectural Archive. Bernadette Goslin's unpublished Master's thesis remains the most invaluable guide to the Murray Collection. The Irish Architectural Archive also contains series of historic photographs – contained in box files and catalogued according to street – of key buildings and urban spaces in Dublin including images of the Westmoreland Lock Hospital (Townsend Street) and the Rotunda (Parnell Street). The box file for the latter also contains photographs of the drawings presented to the marquis of Buckingham in 1788, the originals of which are contained in the British Library, London. Another photographic collection of urban scenes (including depictions of Monto in the early twentieth century) is contained in the Dublin City Archive on Pearse Street.

The Architectural Archive of Ireland also contains hard copies of the *Irish Builder and Engineer* vols 1–72, 1856–1930, whose series entitled 'History of Dublin Hospitals and Infirmaries from 1188 till the Present Time', 1896–97 and, 'Old Dublin Mansion Houses: their lordly occupants in the century', 1894, provided not only a good source of reference but also gave an enlightening indication of the breadth of subjects that came under a nineteenth-century architect/engineer's remit as well as their attitudes towards urban space and indeed, social phenomena. The library at the School of Architecture, University College Dublin at Richview contains a microfiche set of the same publication as well as copies of many of the maps used to illustrate this book. A hard copy of the first edition of the Ordnance Survey of Ireland can be found in the Special Collections at University College Dublin library at Belfield.

Eighteenth-century periodicals and newspapers such as *Dublin Evening Post*, *Hibernian Journal*, *Faulkner's Dublin Journal* and *Hibernian Magazine* etc. were also instructive in providing specific details as well as a flavour of urban life in the Dublin of that time. Many of these are contained in the Newspaper Collection on microfiche at the National Library of Ireland on Kildare Street. Also contained here are hard copies of guides to the city such as Watson's *Gentleman and Citizen's Almanack*. Published throughout the eighteenth century, the latter proved an invaluable source of often quite detailed information concerning the medical institutions of Dublin and their governors as well as lists and other information (including sometimes addresses) of the licensed physicians, surgeons, apothecaries and obstetricians who were working in the city. Other guides to Dublin contained in the National Library include Warburton, Whitelaw and Walsh's *History of the City of Dublin* (1818); Wright's *An Historical Guide to the City of Dublin* (1821); and Curry's *The New Picture of Dublin or, Stranger's Guide through the Irish Metropolis* (1841). These provide a snapshot of the city in the early nineteenth century and include often quite candid descriptions of key buildings and institutions and their functions, ranging from the magnificent Custom House to the decrepit and squalid Newgate Gaol. Also contained in the National Library are Frank Duff's observations on the last days of Monto which can be found in bound volumes of *Maria Legionis: the Organ of the Legion of Mary, 1939–41*. The National Library also contains original copies of some of the key texts concerning nineteenth-century prostitution including Parent-Duchâtelet's *De la prostitution dans la ville de Paris* (1837) and Logan's *The Great Social Evil: its causes and remedies* (1871) as well as Mayhew's *London Labour and the London Poor* (1862). Finally, the Pamphlet Collection of the same institution contains a great deal of material relating to the Lying-in Hospital, Rotunda and Assembly Rooms including, for example, some accounts and registers, a copy of the Royal Charter and the sermon intended to have been preached in the chapel by the Revd Lawson.

Ackermann, J.S. (1966) *Palladio*, London: Penguin.
Acton, W. (1857, 1870) *Prostitution: considered in its moral, social and sanitary aspects in London and other large cities and garrison towns with proposals for the control and prevention of its attendant evils*. London. Reprinted by Frank Cass, London, (1972).
Aheron, J. (1754) *A treatise on architecture in five books*. Dublin.
Anonymous (attributed to William Jebb) (1771) *View of the schemes at present under consideration of the governors of the Lying-in Hospital, Dublin*. Dublin: National Library of Ireland.
Alsayyad, N. (1992) *Forms of dominance: on the architecture and urbanism of the colonial enterprise*. Aldershot: Avebury.
Archdall, M. (1786) *Monasticon Hibernicum, or, A history of the abbeys, priories, and other religious houses in Ireland*. Reprinted (1876) Dublin: W.B. Kelly.
Barret, R M. (1884) *Guide to Dublin charities, vols. 1–3*. Dublin.
Bartlett, T. and Jeffrey, K. (eds) (1996) *A military history of Ireland*. Cambridge: Cambridge University Press.
Betjeman, J. (1951) Francis Johnston: Irish architect. *In*: Evans, M. (ed.) *The pavilion: a contemporary collection of British art and architecture*, London: IT Publications, pp 21–38.
Bender, J. (1987) *Imagining the penitentiary: fiction and the architecture of mind in eighteenth century England*. Chicago: University of Chicago Press.
Benjamin, W. (1935) Paris, the capital of the nineteenth century. *In*: Benjamin, W. (trans. Eiland, H. and McLaughlin, K.) (1999) *The Arcades Project*. Cambridge, MA: Belknap Press, pp 3–13.
Benjamin, W. (1939) Paris, capital of the nineteenth century. *In*: Benjamin, W. (trans. Eiland, H. and McLaughlin, K., 1999) *The Arcades Project*. Cambridge, MA: Belknap Press, pp 14–26.
Berke, D. and Harris, S. (eds) (1997) *Architecture of the everyday*. New York: Princeton Architectural Press.
Berman, M. (1983) *All that's solid melts into air: the experience of modernity*. London: Verso.
Berresford, E.P. (ed.) (1988) *James Connolly: selected writings*. London: Pluto Press.
Bindman, D. (1981) *Hogarth*. London: Thames and Hudson.
Boyd, G.A. (2000) Erosion: closed circuit mapping in Temple Bar, Dublin, *Tracings*, vol. 1. Dublin, pp 110–11.
Boyd, G.A. (2002) Conceits and misconceptions: medicine, monumentality and myth, Dublin 1745–1922. Unpublished PhD thesis. Dublin: University College Dublin.
Boyd, G.A. (2002) Legitimising the illicit: Dublin's Temple Bar and the Monto, *Tracings*, vol. 2. Dublin, pp 112–25.
Boyd, G.A. (2003) Spectacle and myth in O'Connell/Sackville Street, Dublin, *RANAM: recherches anglaises et nord-américaines*, 36. Strasbourg, pp 101–11.
Boydell, B. (1992) *Rotunda music in eighteenth-century Dublin*. Dublin: Irish Academic Press.
Boydell, B. (1988) *A Dublin musical calendar: 1700–1760*. Dublin: Irish Academic Press.
Boyer, M.C. (1996) *City of collective memory: its historical imagery and architectural entertainments*. Cambridge, MA: M.I.T. Press.
Brady, C. (1854) *The practicability of improving the dwellings of the labouring classes with remarks on the law of settlement and removal of the poor*. London.
Brady C. (1865) *The history of the hospital for incurables*. Dublin.
Brady J. and Simms A. (eds) (2001) *Dublin through space and time*. Dublin: Four Courts Press.
Bristow, E. (1977) *Vice and vigilance: purity movements in Britain since 1700*. Dublin: Gill and MacMillan.
Bristowe, J.S. and Holmes, T. (1864) Report on the hospitals of the United Kingdom, *British Parliamentary Papers*, xxxviii.

Browne, A. (ed.) (1995) *Masters, midwives and ladies in waiting: the Rotunda Hospital, 1745–1995.* Dublin: Governors of the Rotunda Hospital.

Browne, O.T.D. (1947) *The Rotunda Hospital, 1744–1945.* Edinburgh: E. and S. Livingstone.

Bullough, B. and Bullough, V. (1987) *Women and prostitution: a social history.* Buffalo, NY: Prometheus Books.

Burke, H. (1993) *The Royal Hospital, Donnybrook: a heritage of caring.* Dublin: The Royal Hospital Donnybrook and the Social Science Research Centre, University College Dublin.

Buck-Morss, S. (1989) *The dialectics of seeing: Walter Benjamin and the Arcades Project.* Cambridge, MA: M.I.T. Press.

Bush, J. (1764) *Hibernia Curiosa.* London.

Campbell, H. (1998) Contested territory, common ground. Dublin: unpublished PhD thesis, University College Dublin.

Campbell-Ross, I. (ed.) (1986) *Public virtue, public love: the early years of the Dublin Lying-in Hospital, the Rotunda.* Dublin: O'Brien Press.

Capuchin Annual (1932–4). Dublin.

Cappock, M. (2000) Pageantry or propaganda? *The Illustrated London News* and royal visitors in Ireland, GPA, *Irish Arts Review Yearbook.* Dublin, pp 86–93.

Caulfield, M. (1995) *The Easter rebellion.* Dublin: Gill and Macmillan.

Celik, Z., Favro, D. and Ingersoll, R. (eds) (1994) *Streets: critical perspectives on public space.* Los Angeles: University of California Press.

Chambers, W. (1759) *A treatise on civil architecture.* London.

Clarke, H. (ed.) (1990) Medieval Dublin: *the making of a metropolis.* Dublin: Irish Academic Press, Dublin.

Collum, W. (1770) *Reasons against lectures in the Lying-in Hospital.* Dublin.

Colomina B. (ed.) (1992) *Sexuality and space.* New York: Princeton Architectural Press.

Colomina, B. (1997) The medical body in modern architecture, *Daidalos,* 64. Berlin, pp 60–71.

Connolly, J. (1910) *Labour in Irish history.* Reprinted by New Books, Dublin (1983).

Connolly, J. (1910) *Labour, nationality and religion.* Reprinted by New Books, Dublin (1983).

Connolly, J. (1910) *The re-conquest of Ireland.* Reprinted by New Books, Dublin (1983).

Connolly, J. (1915) Insurrectionary warfare, *The Workers' Republic,* May-July, 1915.

Conroy, E. (1997) No rest for twenty years. Dublin: unpublished MA thesis, University College Dublin.

Cope, H. (1737) *Medicine vindicata: or Reflections of bleeding, vomitting and purging in the beginning of fevers, small-pox, pleurisie and other acute diseases.* London.

Cosgrove, D.E. (1993) *The Palladian landscape: its geographical change and its cultural representation in sixteenth-century Italy.* Leicester: Leicester University Press.

Craig, M. (1992) *Dublin, 1660–1860.* London: Penguin.

Craig, M. (1948) *The volunteer earl: being the life and times of James Caulfeild, first earl of Charlemont.* London.

Croker King, S. (1785) *A short history of the hospital founded by Dr Richard Steevens.* Dublin.

Cullen, F. (1997) *Visual politics: the representation of Ireland, 1750–1930.* Cork: Cork University Press.

Cullen, M.J. (1975) *The statistical movement in early Victorian Britain: the foundation of empirical social research.* New York: Harvester Press.

Curran, C.P. (1947) *The Rotunda Hospital: its architects and craftsmen.* Dublin: Three Candles.

Curriculum Development Unit, Dublin (1978) *Divided city: portrait of Dublin, 1913.* Dublin: O'Brien Educational.

Curry, W. (1841) *The new picture of Dublin or Stranger's guide through the Irish metropolis.* Dublin.

Daly, M.E. (1984) *Dublin: the deposed capital: a social and economic history, 1860–1914.* Cork: Cork University Press.

Dalsimer, A. D. (1993) *Visualising Ireland: national identity and the pictorial tradition*, London: Faber and Faber.
Davis, M. (1990) *The city of quartz*. London: Random House.
Dennis, M. (1986) *Court and garden: from the French hôtel to the city of modern architecture*. Cambridge, MA: M.I.T. Press.
Dickson, D. (2000) *New foundation: Ireland, 1600–1800*. Dublin: Irish Academic Press.
Dickson, D. (ed.) (1987) *The gorgeous mask: Dublin, 1700–1850*. Dublin: Trinity History Workshop Group.
Donnison, J. (1977) *Midwives and medical men: A history of inter-professional rivalries and women's rights*. London: Heinemann.
Douglas, M. (1996) *Purity and danger: an analysis of the concepts of pollution and taboo*. London: Routledge.
Dublin Hospital Reports and Communications in Medicine and Surgery (1817–1830). 5 vols. Dublin.
Durning, L. and Wigley, R. (eds) (2000) *Gender and architecture*. Chichester: John Wiley and Son.
Eagleton, T. (1991) *Ideology: an introduction*. London: Verso.
Evans, R. (1982) *The fabrication of virtue, English prison architecture, 1750–1840*, Cambridge: Cambridge University Press.
Fagan, T. (2000) *Monto: madams, murder and black coddle*. Dublin: North Inner City Folk History Project.
Finnegan, F. (2001) *Do penance or perish: a study of Magdalen asylums in Ireland*. Kilkenny: Congrave Press.
Finzsch, N. and Jütte, R. (eds) (1996) *Institutions of confinement: hospitals, asylums and prisons in Western Europe and North America, 1500–1900*. Cambridge: Cambridge University Press.
Fitzgerald, B. (1957) *Correspondence of Emily, duchess of Kildare, 1731–1814*, Dublin: Stationery Office.
Fitzmaurice, Lord E. (1875) *William, earl of Shelburne*. London.
Fleetwood, J.F. (1988) *The Irish body snatchers: a history of body snatching in Ireland*. Dublin: Tomar Publishing.
Fleetwood, J.F. (1951) *The history of medicine in Ireland*. Dublin. Reprinted by Brown and Nolan. Dublin, (1983).
Forster, K.W., (1977) Stagecraft and statecraft: the architectural integration of public life and theatrical spectacle in Scamozzi's theater at Sabbioneta, *Oppositions*, 9. Cambridge, MA. pp 63–89.
Forty, A. (1980) The modern hospital in England and France: the social and medical uses of architecture. *In*: King, A.D. (ed.) *Buildings and society: essays on the social development of the built environment*. London: Routledge and Kegan Paul, pp 61–78.
Foster, R.F. (1988) *Modern Ireland, 1600–1972*. London: Penguin Books.
Foucault, M. (2000) *The birth of the clinic: an archaeology of medical perception*. London: Routledge.
Foucault, M. (1977) *Discipline and punish: the birth of the prison*. London: Penguin Books.
Foucault, M. (1993) *Madness and civilisation: a history of insanity in the age of reason*. London: Routledge.
Foster, E. (1768) *An essay on hospitals or, Succinct directions for the situation, construction and administration of country hospitals*. Dublin.
Foy, M. and Barton, B. (eds) (1999) *The Easter rising*. London: Sutton Publishing.
Fraser, M. (1985) Public building and colonial policy in Dublin, 1760–1800, *Architectural History*, 28, pp 102–22.

Fraser, M. (1996) *John Bull's other homes: state housing and British policy in Ireland, 1883–1922*. Liverpool: Liverpool University Press.
Fyffe, N.R. (ed.) (1998) *Images of the street: planning, identity and control in public space*. London: Routledge.
Gatenby, P. (1996) *Dublin's Meath Hospital, 1753–1996*. Dublin: Townhouse.
Gilbert, J.T. (ed.) (1899–1944) *Calendar of the ancient records of Dublin in possession of the municipal corporation*. 19 vols, Dublin: Joseph Dollard.
Gillespie, R. and Kennedy, B.P. (1994) *Ireland: art in history*. Dublin: Townhouse.
Goold, G.P. (ed.) (1987) *Vitruvius on architecture*. Cambridge, MA: Harvard University Press, 1987.
Goslin, B. (1990) A history and descriptive catalogue of the Murray collection of architectural drawings in the collection of the Royal Institute of Architects of Ireland. Dublin: unpublished MA thesis, University College Dublin.
Griffin, D.J. and Pegum, C. (2000) *Leinster House, 1744–2000: an architectural history*. Dublin: Irish Architectural Archive.
Guinness, D. (1979) *Georgian Dublin*. London: Batsford.
Haliday C. (1884) *The Scandinavian kingdom of Dublin*, London.
Harbison, P. (ed.) (1991) *Beranger's views of Ireland*. Dublin: Royal Irish Academy.
Harvey, D. (1985) *The urban experience*. London: Blackwell.
Harvey, D. (1990) *The condition of post-modernity*, London: Blackwell.
Henry, B. (1994) *Dublin hanged: crime, law enforcement and punishment in late eighteenth-century Dublin*. Dublin: Irish Academic Press.
Hobson, B. (1918) *A short history of the Irish Volunteers*. Dublin.
Howard, J. (1791) *An account of the principal lazarettos in Europe; with various papers relative to the Plague: Together with further observations on some foreign hospitals and prisons; and additional remarks on the present state of those in Great Britain and Ireland*. London.
Igoe, V. and O'Dwyer, F. (1988) Early views of the Royal Hospital, Kilmainham, *GPA Irish Arts Review Yearbook*. Dublin, pp 78–88.
Jackson, P. (1998) Domesticating the street: the contested spaces of the high street and the mall. *In*: Fyffe, N.R. (ed.) *Images of the street: planning, identity and control in public space*. London: Routledge, pp 176–91.
Jones, C. (1996) The construction of the hospital patient in early modern France. *In*: Finzsch, N. and Jütte, R. (eds) *Institutions of confinement: hospitals, asylums and prisons in Western Europe and North America, 1500–1900*. Cambridge: Cambridge University Press, pp 55–74.
Jones, G. and Malcolm, E. (eds) (1991) *Medicine, disease and the state in Ireland, 1640–1940*. Cork: Cork University Press.
Joyce, J. (1922) *Ulysses*. Reprinted by Penguin Books, London, (1992).
Joyce, J. (1916) *Portrait of the artist as a young man*. Reprinted by Paladin, London (1988).
Joyce, J. (1944) *Stephen Hero*. Reprinted by Paladin, London (1991).
Kiberd, D. (2001) *Irish classics*. London: Granta Books.
King, A.D. (ed.) (1980) *Buildings and society: essays on the social development of the built environment*. London: Routledge and Kegan Paul.
Kirkpatrick, T.P. (1924) *The history of Dr Steevens' Hospital, Dublin, 1720–1920*. Dublin.
Kirkpatrick, T.P. (1933) *The foundation of a great hospital: Steevens' in the XVIIIth century*. Dublin.
Kirkpatrick, T.P. and Jellet, H. (1914) *The book of the Rotunda Hospital: an illustrated history of the Dublin lying-in hospital from its foundation to the present time*. London.
La Tocnaye, Le Chevalier de (1801) *A Frenchman's walk through Ireland, 1796–7*. Reprinted by Blackstaff Press, London (1984).

Landreth, H. (1949) *The pursuit of Robert Emmet*. Dublin.
Lawson, Revd J. (1759) *A sermon intended to have been preached at the public opening of the chappel of the lying-in hospital in Great Britain-street, Dublin*. Dublin: National Library of Ireland.
Lee, G. (1996) *Leper hospitals in medieval Ireland*. Dublin: Four Courts Press.
Lefebvre, H. (1991) *The production of space*. Oxford: Blackwell.
Lefebvre, H. (1996) *Writings on cities*, Oxford: Blackwell.
Levenson, S. (1973) *James Connolly: a biography*. London: Martin, Brian and O'Keefe.
Llanover, Lady (ed.) (1926) *Mrs. Delaney: at court and among the wits: being the record of a great lady, arranged from the autobiography and correspondence of Mrs Delany with interesting reminiscences of George III and Queen Charlotte*. London.
Logan, W. (1871) *The great social evil: its causes, extents, results and remedies*. London.
Luddy, M. and Murphy, C. (eds) (1990) *Women surviving*. Dublin: Poolbeg Press.
Lyons, J.B. (1991) *The quality of Mercer's: the story of Mercer's Hospital*. Dublin: Glendale Publishing.
Lyons, M. (ed.) (1995) *The memoirs of Mrs Leeson, Madam, 1727–1797*. Dublin: Lilliput Press.
Malcolm, E. (1989) *Swift's hospital: a history of St Patrick's Hospital, Dublin, 1746–1989*. Dublin: Gill and MacMillan.
Malcolm, E. and Jones, G. *Medicine, disease and the state in Ireland, 1650–1940*. Cork: Cork University Press.
Malton, J. (1799) *A picturesque and descriptive view of the city of Dublin*. Reprinted by Dolmen Press, Dublin, 1978.
Markus, T.A. (1993) *Buildings and power: freedom and control in the origin of the modern building type*. London: Routledge.
Mayhew, H. (1862) *London labour and the London poor; volume III: those that will not work – comprising prostitutes, swindlers, thieves and beggars*. London.
McAvoy, S. (1999) The regulation of sexuality in the Irish Free State. *In*: Malcolm, E. and Jones, G. *Medicine, disease and the state in Ireland, 1650–1940*. Cork: Cork University Press.
McBride, L.W. (ed.) (1999) *Images, icons and the Irish nationalist imagination*. Dublin: Four Courts Press.
McCullough, N. (1989) *Dublin: an urban history*. Dublin: Anne St Press.
McDonagh, O. (1983) *States of mind: a study of the Anglo-Irish conflict, 1780–1980*. London: George Allan and Unwin.
McHugh, P. (1980) *Prostitution and Victorian social reform*. London: Croom Helm.
McCready, C.T. (1892) *Street names dated and explained*. Reprinted by Carraig Book, Dublin, (1987).
McLeod, M. (1997) Henri Lefebvre's Critique of everyday life: an introduction. *In*: Berke, D. and Harris, S. (eds) *Architecture of the Everyday*. New York: Princeton Architectural Press, pp 9–29.
McParland, E. (1969) Francis Johnston, architect, 1760–1829, *Bulletin of the Irish Georgian Society*, 12 (2), pp 62–139.
McParland, E. (1972) The Wide Streets Commissioners: their importance for Dublin architecture in the late 18th and early 19th Century, *Bulletin of the Irish Georgian Society*, 15 (1), pp 1–32.
McParland, E. (2001) *Public architecture in Ireland, 1680–1760*. New Haven; London: Yale University Press.
Middleton, R. (1994) Sickness, madness and crime as the grounds of form, part 1, *AA Files*, 24. London, pp 16–30.

Middleton, R. (1994) Sickness, madness and crime as the grounds of form, part 2, *AA Files*, 25. London, pp 14–29.
Moorehead, T.G. (1942) *A short history of Patrick Dun's hospital*. Dublin.
Murphy, T.W. (1916) *The Sinn Fein Rebellion: Dublin the six days' rebellion, thirty-one pictures from the camera of Mr T.W. Murphy*. Dublin.
Neale, R.S. (1981) *Bath, 1680–1850: a social history, or, a valley of pleasure, yet a sink of iniquity*. London: Routledge and Kegan Paul.
O'Brien, E. (ed.) (1987) *The charitable infirmary, Jervis Street, 1718–1987: a farewell tribute*. Dublin: Anniversary Press.
O'Brien, E., Crookshank, A. and Wolstenholme, G.A. (1984) *A portrait of Irish medicine*. Dublin: Ward River Press.
O'Casey, S. (1985) *Plays by Sean O'Casey*. Edited by R. Ayling, London: MacMillan.
O'Connor, J. (1995) *The workhouses of Ireland: the fate of Ireland's Poor*, Dublin: Anvil Books.
O'Connor, C. (1999) *The pleasing hours: James Caulfeild, first earl of Charlemont, 1728–99, traveller, connoisseur and patron of the arts in Ireland*. Cork: Collins Press.
O'Donal Brown, T.D. (1947) *The Rotunda Hospital, 1745–1945*. Edinburgh.
O'Dwyer, F. (1981) *Lost Dublin*. Dublin: Gill and MacMillan.
O'Dwyer, F. (1997) *Irish hospital architecture: a pictorial history*. Dublin: Department of Health and Children.
Ogborn, M. (1998) *Spaces of modernity: London's geographies, 1680–1780*. New York: Guildford Press.
O'Grady, S. (1880) *History of Ireland, volume 2: Cuculainn and his contemporaries*. Dublin.
O'Kane, F. (2000) Mixing foreign trees with the natives: Irish demesne landscape in the eighteenth century. Dublin: unpublished PhD thesis, University College Dublin.
O'Kane, F. (2000) Nurturing a revolution: Patrick Pearse's school gardens at St Enda's, *Journal of Garden History*, 28 (1), pp 73–87.
Olley, J. (1990) 20 St James's Square, Part 1, *Architects' Journal*, 8, pp 34–57.
Olley, J. (1990) 20 St James's Square, Part 2, *Architects' Journal*, 9, pp 34–53.
Olley, J. (1992) Sustaining the narrative at Kilmainham, *GPA Irish Arts Review Yearbook*, Dublin, pp 65–72.
Olley, J. (1993) The theatre of the city: Dublin, 1991, *GPA Irish Arts Review Yearbook*, Dublin, pp 70–8.
O'Regan, J. (ed.) (1998) *A monument in the city: Nelson's Pillar*. Dublin: Gandon Editions.
O'Snodaigh, A. (1996) *The Rotunda: birthplace of the Irish Volunteers*. Dublin: Republican News.
Outram, D. (1995) *The Enlightenment*. Cambridge: Cambridge University Press.
Pallasmaa, J. (1996) *The eyes of the skin: architecture and the senses*. London: Polemics: Academy Editions.
Papworth, W. (ed.) (1852–92) *The dictionary of architecture*. 8 vols. London: Architecture Publication Society.
Parent-Duchâtelet, A.J.B. (1837) *De la prostitution dans la ville de Paris*. London.
Pearse, P.H. (undated) *Collected works: political writings and speeches*. Dublin.
Pearse, P.H. (1917) *Collected works: plays, stories, poems*. Dublin.
Pearse, P.H. and Ryan, D. (eds) (1920) *The story of a success: being a record of St Enda's College, September 1908 to Easter 1916*, Dublin.
Peter, A. (1925) *Dublin fragments*. Dublin: Hodges Figgis.
Peter, A. (1907) *A brief account of the Magdalen Chapel, Lower Leeson Street, Dublin*. Dublin.
Peter, A. (1907) *Sketches of Old Dublin*. Dublin.
Pevsner, N. (1976) *A history of building types*. London: Thames and Hudson.

Pile, S. (1996) *The body and the city*. London: Routledge.
Pool, R. and Cash, J. (1780) *Views of the most remarkable public buildings, monuments and other edifices in the city of Dublin*. Dublin.
Porter, R. (1994) *London: a social history*. London: Hamish Hamilton.
Prunty, J. (1998) *Dublin slums, 1800–1925: a study of urban geography*. Dublin: Irish Academic Press.
Quétel, C. (1990) *History of syphillis*. Cambridge: Polity Press.
Rabinow, P. (ed.) (1991) *A Foucault reader: an introduction to Foucault's thought*, London: Penguin.
Reynolds, M. (1983) *A history of the Irish Post Office*. Dublin: McDonnell Whyte.
Ryan, L. (1997) *Reading the prostitute: appearance, place and time in British and Irish press stories of prostitution*. London: Ashgate Press.
Said, E.W. (1994) *Culture and imperialism*. London: Vintage.
Sante, L. (1991) *Low-life: drinking, drugging, whoring, murder, corruption, vice and miscellaneous mayhem in old New York*. London: Granta.
Schlör, J. (1998) *Nights in the big city*. London: Reaktion Books.
Scobie, A. (1990) *Hitler's state architecture: the impact of Classical antiquity*. London: published for College Art Association by Pennsylvania State University Press.
Semple, G. (1780) *Hibernia's free trade*. Dublin.
Sennett, R. (1990) *The conscience of the eye*. London: Faber and Faber.
Sennett, R. (1977) *The fall of public man*. Cambridge: Cambridge University Press.
Sennett, R. (1994) *Flesh and stone: the body and the city in Western society*. London: Norton.
Serlio, S. (1611) *The five books of architecture*. Unabridged reprint of the English edition of 1611, Dover Publications, New York, (1982).
Shaffrey, M. (1988) Sackville Street/O'Connell Street, *GPA Irish Arts Review Yearbook*, Dublin, pp 144–56.
Shaw, H. (1850) *The Dublin pictorial guide and directory of 1850*. Reprinted by Friar's Bush Press, Dublin, (1988).
Sibley, D. (1995) *Geographies of exclusion*. London: Routledge.
Solkin, D.H. (1982) *Richard Wilson: the landscape of reaction*. London: Tate Gallery.
Solkin, D.H. (1993) *Painting for money: the visual arts and the public sphere in eighteenth-century England*. London: Yale University Press.
Spongberg, M. (1997) *The body of the prostitute in nineteenth-century medical discourse*. London: MacMillan Press, 1997.
Stafford, B.A. (1993) *Body criticism: imaging the unseen in Enlightenment art and medicine*. Cambridge, MA: M.I.T. Press.
Stevenson, C. (2000) *Medicine and magnificence: British hospital and asylum architecture, 1660–1815*. London: Yale University Press.
Strong, R. (1984) *Art and power*, London: Boydell Press.
Summerson, J. (1986) *The architecture of the eighteenth century*. London: Thames and Hudson.
Summerson, J. (1993) *The Classical language of architecture*. London: Thames and Hudson.
Sumption, J. (1975) *Pilgrimage: an image of mediaeval religion*. London: Faber and Faber.
Tafuri, M. (1976) *Architecture and utopia*. Cambridge, MA: M.I.T. Press.
Tavernor, R. (1991) *Palladio and Palladianism*. London: Thames and Hudson.
Taylor, J. (1991) *Hospital and asylum architecture in England, 1840–1914*. London: Mansell Publishing.
Taylor, R. (1984) *A reader's guide to the plays of W.B. Yeats*. London: MacMillan Press.
Thompson, J.D. and Goldin, G. (1975) *The hospital: a social and architectural history*. London: Yale University Press.

Thompson, W.I.(1967) *The imagination of an insurrection: Dublin, Easter 1916, a study of an ideological movement*. Oxford: Oxford University Press.

Tilllyard, S. (1995) *Aristocrats: Caroline, Emily, Louisa and Sarah Lennox, 1740–1832*. London: Vintage.

Todd, C.H. (1818) *Surgical report containing an account of those fections of the penis which are generally considered as primary symptoms of syphilis, with the modes of treatment employed in the Richmond Hospital*. Dublin Hospital Reports in Medicine and Surgery.

Tone, T.W. (1791) *An argument on behalf of the Catholics of Ireland*. Dublin.

Turpin, J. (2000) *Oliver Sheppard (1865–1941): symbolic sculptor of the Irish cultural revival*. Dublin: Four Courts Press.

Walkowitz, J.R. (1980) *Prostitution and Victorian society: women, class and the state*. Cambridge: Cambridge University Press.

Walkowitz, J. R. (1992) *Cities of dreadful delight: narratives of sexual danger in late Victorian London*. Chicago: University of Chicago Press.

Warburton, J., Whitelaw, J. and Walsh R. (1818) *The history of the city of Dublin: from the earliest accounts to the present time*. 2 vols. London.

Ward, M. (1983) *Unmanageable revolutionaries: women and Irish nationalism*. London: Pluto Press.

Weisman, L.K. (1994) *Discrimination by design*. Chicago: University of Illinois Press.

Whelan, Y. (2003) *Reinventing modern Dublin: streetscape, iconography and the politics of identity*. Dublin: University College Dublin Press.

White, J. (undated) *The Rotunda: or characteristic sketches of the speakers at the religious meetings held there*. Dublin: National Library of Ireland.

Wilde, W. (1846) Illustrious physicians and surgeons in Ireland: Bartholomew Mosse M.D., surgeon, *Dublin Quarterly of Medical Science*, II, Dublin: National Library of Ireland, pp 566–96.

Williams, D.I. (1988) *The London Lock: a charitable hospital for venereal disease, 1746–1952*. London: Royal Society of Medicine Press.

Williams, R. (1985) *The country and the city*. London: Hogarth Press.

Williams, R. (1988) *Keywords*. London: Fontana Press.

Wilson, E. (1991) *The sphinx in the city: urban life, the control of disorder and women*, Oxford: University of California Press.

Wilton-Ely, J. (1978) *The mind and art of Giovanni Battista Piranesi*, London: Thames and Hudson.

Wölfflinn, H. (1952) *Classic art: an introduction to the Italian Renaissance*. Reprinted by Phaidon Press, London (1994).

Wollstonecraft, M. (1792) *Vindication of the rights of Women*. Reprinted by Penguin Books and edited by M. Brody, London (1992).

Wollstonecraft, M. (1798) *Mary, a fiction and the wrongs of women*. Reprinted by Oxford University Press and edited by G. Kelly London (1976).

Wolveridge, J. (1671) *Speculum Matricis Hibernicum*. London.

Wright, G.N. (1825) *An historic guide to the city of Dublin*. London.

Yeats, W.B. (1934) *Collected plays*. London: Gill and Macmillan.

Yeats, W.B. (1938) *Collected poems*. London: Gill and Macmillan.

Zukin, S. (1991) *Landscapes of power*. Los Angeles: University of California Press.

Illustrations

1	Portrait of Bartholomew Mosse.	14
2	Locations of old and new Lying-in Hospital.	15
3	Locations of Hospitals in Dublin in 1745.	17
4	The Charitable Infirmary on Inn's Quay.	19
5	Mercer's Hospital.	19
6	The Poor House (later Foundling Hospital).	19
7	The Royal Hospital, Kilmainham.	20
8	Steeven's Hospital.	21
9	The original Lying-in Hospital building.	28
10	The locale of the original Lying-in Hospital at George's Lane.	29
11	The cover of John Blunt's *Man-Midwifery Dissected*.	30
12	Portrait of James and Emily, earl and countess of Kildare.	35
13	Kildare House west front.	41
14	Plan of Kildare House and Gardens on the eastern fringes of the city.	42
15	Kildare House west elevation.	44
16	Front façade of the Lying-in Hospital.	44
17	Plan of the Lying-in Hospital in its urban context.	45
18	'Taste, à-la-mode 1745'.	47
19	Interior of Theatre Royal, 1795.	48
20	Sackville Street and Mall.	49
21	Royal Hospital and Ranelagh Gardens, London.	51
22	City Bason.	52
23	Marlborough Bowling Green.	52
24	Lottery ticket displaying the Lying-in Hospital elevation.	56
25	Kildare House, ground floor plan and courtyard.	57
26	The new Lying-in Hospital and gardens.	58
27	Plan of the 'Principal Floor' of the Lying-in Hospital.	61
28	Plan of 'Bed-chamber Floor' of Lying-in Hospital.	62
29	Cross-section of Lying-in Hospital.	62
30	Entrance Hall of the Lying-in Hospital.	64
31	Temple front detail of the Lying-in Hospital's front façade.	67
32	Detail of the Lying-in Hospital chapel: statue of Faith.	69
33	Detail of Lying-in Hospital chapel: statue of Charity.	69
34	Lying-in Hospital chapel viewed from the 'Principal Floor'.	70
35	Long section of Lying-in Hospital.	74
36	Elevation of Charlemont House.	77
37	Charlemont House and its relationship to the Lying-in Hospital and gardens.	78
38	Interior of Rotunda at Ranelagh, London.	80
39	View of the Lying-in Hospital and Rotunda.	81
40	Elevation of Edward Foster's design for a hospital.	84
41	Ground floor plan of Edward Foster's design for a hospital.	84
42	First floor plan of Edward Foster's design for a hospital.	85
43	Plans and elevation of the London Hospital.	89

44	Elevation of the Hospital for Incurables.	90
45	Ground floor plan of St Patrick's Hospital.	91
46	Elevation of St Patrick's Hospital.	91
47	Schematic of James Malton's view of the city of Dublin from the west.	92
48	Plan of the Assembly Rooms, Dublin.	97
49	The Cavendish Row elevation of the Assembly Rooms, Dublin.	98
50	Plan of the Lying-in Hospital, Rotunda and Assembly Rooms.	100
51	View of the completed Assembly Rooms, Dublin.	102
52	View of Charlemont House and the New Pleasure Gardens.	103
53	Elevations of Sackville Street extension executed under Wide Streets Commissioners.	107
54	Plan of eastern Dublin in 1780 before the extension of Sackville Street to the river.	108
55	Plan of eastern Dublin after Sackville Street's extension.	109
56	View of the Royal Exchange from Capel Street.	114
57	View of temple front of the Assembly Rooms.	114
58	Plan of Dublin with the interventions of the Wide Streets Commissioners highlighted.	116
59	View of the Royal Exchange.	117
60	Elevation of Newgate Gaol, Dublin.	118
61	View of Newgate Gaol, London.	118
62	Debtor's Door at Newgate Gaol, London.	119
63	Detail of façade at Newgate Gaol, Dublin.	119
64	'Taste-à-la-mode, 1790'.	125
65	Extracts from the Lying-in Hospital Patient Register, 1745.	130
66	Extracts from the Lying-in Hospital Patient Register, 1791.	130
67	Lying-in admission certificate.	132
68	The Doric, Ionic, Corinthian orders.	135
69	View of Corinthian column in the Lying-in Hospital chapel.	136
70	Interior of the Magdalen Asylum chapel in Leeson Street, Dublin.	138
71	Leeson Street Magdalen Asylum.	140
72	The Lock Penitentiary (Bethesda) near Rutland Square.	141
73	The locations of the Lock Hospital, Dublin, 1755–92.	146
74	The Hospital for Incurables on Lazers Hill.	151
75	Ground floor plan of the Hospital for Incurables.	153
76	Elevation of Hospital for Incurables, Lazers Hill.	155
77	Ground floor plan of the Westmoreland Lock Hospital.	156
78	Plan of the *Ospedale Maggiore*, Milan.	157
79	Plan of Cork Street Fever Hospital.	159
80	Plan of the Royal Military Infirmary.	160
81	Ground floor plan of the Westmoreland Lock Hospital, showing alterations by Francis Johnston.	166
82	View of the Westmoreland Lock Hospital.	167
83	Interior of an unidentified Magdalen Asylum in Ireland.	170
84	Plan of the Westmoreland Lock Hospital in 1847.	171
85	Plan of the Government Lock Hospital at Kildare.	172
86	Ground floor plan of the Richmond Penitentiary.	175
87	'Cease to Do Evil Gate', Richmond House of Correction.	176

ILLUSTRATIONS 219

88	Plan showing location of Monto.	177
89	Plan of Monto in 1837.	178
90	Elliot Place in Monto.	188
91	Faithful Place in Monto.	189
92	Plan of Monto in the 1930s.	192
93	Sackville Street from Carlisle Bridge in the early nineteenth century.	195
94	Tragic theatre set by Sebastiano Serlio.	195
95	Elevation of the General Post Office.	196
96	Elevation of Sackville Street, 1850.	198

Index

Page numbers in italic refer to illustrations; in bold, to sections of chapters.

Abercromby, Sir Ralph 143
absenteeism 163
abuse, physical 129
access, hospital 59, 64, 83, 156–7, 158
accommodation, servants 57, 58
Account of the principle Lazarettos of Europe 155
Act of Union 142, 145, 174, 181, 191
Acton, William *Prostitution: Considered in its Moral, Social and Sanitary Aspects* 184, 185
Acts of parliament 37, 82, 103, 104–5, 115, 123, 142, 169, 179
Adam, James 101
Adam, Richard 101
Adam, Robert 40
admissions procedure 59, **129–34**, 145–6, 163–4
advertising 54, 56, 101, 197
agricultural changes 38, 199
Aheron, John *A General Treatise of Architecture in Five Books* 135–6
Alberti, Leon Battista 110, 112, 120
alcohol 123, 143, 187, 190
Aldborough House 181
Alexander, James 105
ancien régime 17–18, 20, 26, 86, 146, 157, 158, 165
Anglo-Irish 16, 37–9, 66, 198, 201. *see also* Protestantism
Archdall, Mervyn *Monasticum Hibernicum* 94
architecture. *see also* façades, building; Palladian architecture
  Assembly Rooms **96–9**, *100*, *101–2*, 113–14
  big houses 36, 37, **40–6, 56–8,** 78
  circular system 157–8, 165
  gaols **116–20,** 174–6
  Hospital for Incurables 90, 153–4, 155, 173
  Lying-in Hospital **27–9, 43–6,** 58, 60–1, *62*, 64, 67, 74, *81*, *100*
  pavilion plan **157–60**
  Westmoreland Lock Hospital **155–60, 162–7,** *171*
aristocracy 35, 48, 55, 56, 112, 121
  sexual pleasures **124–9,** 133
Armagh, archbishop of (George Stone) 34
army. *see* military
Arran, Lord 99
arrests 179, 180, 187
Assembly Rooms **95–103,** 111, 113, *114*, 122, *125*, 142
  architecture 96–9, *100*, 101–2, 113–14
  drawings 96–8, 101
  funding 96, 97, 99–100, 101, 102–3, 104

Association for the Discountenancing of Vice, and Promoting the Knowledge and Practice of the Christian Religion 142
asylums, magdalen **137–40,** 141, *170*, 191
Aughrim, Battle of 54
authority, abuse of 134

ball, masked 126, *127*, 128
Barrack Street 178, 179
Bate, Thomas 93
Bayley, Dean 137–8
Beardsley, Dr 159
Bective, earl of (Thomas Taylour) 99, 128
bed capacity and costs 21, 33, 61, 73–4, 76, 88, 155, 162
Bedford, duke of (Lord Lieutenant) 61–3
Bedlam Asylum, Southwark, London 90–3
beggars 197
Benjamin, Walter 198, 199
Bessborough House, County Kilkenny 39
Bethlem Asylum (Bedlam), Southwark, London 90–3
Bethseda chapel **137–40**
Bevan, Reverend William 184–5
bibles 143
big houses 36, 37, **39–46,** 56–8, 77–8
Bluecoat hospital 16, *17, 18*
Blunt, John *Man-Midwifery Dissected* 30–1
body-snatching 24
Boer war 180
Bolger, Charles 128–9
books, suppression of 143
Boyle, Richard (third earl of Burlington) 101
Brady, Dr Cheyne 152
Brady, Mr 129
Brennan, Alexander 45
Bristol, Lord (Frederick Augustus Hervey) 128
British administration 95, 113, 144, 196–7
  funding 65, 75, 76, 79, 102, 111, 162, 168
Brooks, Mrs 128
brothels **126–9,** 141, 142, 178, 179, 186, 190. *see also* prostitution
Buckingham, earl of (Lord Lieutenant) 98, 99, 101
Buckingham, marquis of 101
Buckingham Smallpox Hospital 147
budget, Irish 144
building boom 37, 38–40, 46–7, 107, 108, 111
Burgh, Thomas 93
Burlington, earl of (Richard Boyle) 101
Bury, William 97
Bush, John 106, 194
  Hibernia Curiosa 49–50

Campbell, Colen 38
Capel Street 107, 116
Carlisle Bridge 107, 194
Carton House, County Kildare 39
Cassels, Richard 37, 39, 45–6, 47, 67
Castletown House, County Kildare 37
Catholics 22, 37, 65, 71, 144
Cato (play) 33
Caulfeild, James (earl of Charlemont) 77, 78–9, 95, 96–7, 99, 103, 105, 106
Cavendish Row 77, *125*
Census of Ireland, first 183
Chambers, Sir William *A Treatise on Civil Architecture* 77–8
chanting, female 139
chapels 86
  Bethseda **137–40**
  Lying-in 60–1, *62*, **66–71,** *74*, 87, **134–7**
Charitable Infirmary 16, *17, 19,* 21, 22, 25, 29, 33
charity 55–6, 63, 65, 66, 69
Charlemont, earl of (James Caulfeild) 77, 78–9, 95, 96–7, 99, 103, 105, 106
Charlemont House *77–8, 103*
Charles II, King 50
Chelsea Hospital 50
children 123
  births 24–5, 81–2
  deaths 26, 81–2, 129, 131
  illegitimate 25–6
  maintenance scheme 73, 75
cholera epidemic, Asian 176, 183
circulation system 157–8, 165
Cipriani, Mr 68, 75
City Bason, James's Street 51, *52*, 55
City Marshalsea 120
Clanbrassil, earl of 99
Clarendon Street *146,* 147
Clarke, Joseph 88
Cleghorn, James 129
Clogher, bishop of 66, 75
coat of arms 113, *114,* 196
College Green 109, 115
Collum, William 32, 194
colonial landscape **34–9**
columns. *see* Corinthian Order; Doric Order; Ionic Order
commerce, influence of 121, 197
concerts, music 54, 55, 56, 121
Conolly, William 37
Contagious Diseases Acts 169–70, 179, 191
controversy
  maternity hospital **29–33**
  medical 23–4
Cooley, Thomas 110, 112, 115–17

220

INDEX

Corinthian Order *135–6, 196*
Cork 169
Cork Street Fever Hospital 25, 158–9
Cornwallis, earl of 145
Craig, Maurice 45, 46, 164
Cramillion, Bartholomew 68–9
Crimea War 181
Criminal Law Amendment Act 179–80, 191
Cromwell, Oliver 37
Cuper's (Cupid's) Gardens 15
Curragh, The 169
Currie, Dr 159
Custom House 194
    relocation of 107, 113

Dame Street 107–8, 115
Dance, George 117, 118–19
Darley, Henry 45
Daughters of Charity 146
De Architectura 135
deaths 46, 68, 75–7
    in childbirth 26, 81–2, 129, 131
debt, hospital 65, 75, 76
Delany, Mrs *quote* 54–5, 123
De la Prostitution dans la Ville de Paris (study) 183–4
de la Tocnaye, Chevalier *Promenade d'un Français en Irlande* 79–80
demesne 36–7, 40
Denny, Lady Arabella 137, 139
disciplinary institutions **174–6**. *see also* asylums, magdalen; gaols
disease 64, 83, 152–3, 155, 158, 173, 183, 197
    Acts 169–71
    'incurable' 150–3
    syphilis 165–6, 179
    venereal 64, 128–9, 141, 145–50, 155, 161, **163–5, 167–73**, 179
disorderly conduct, control of 123–4, 199. *see also* surveillance
dissection, practice of medical 23–4
division, social 115–16, 120–1, 134–5
D'Olier Street 107, 108
domestic premises, hospitals in 20–2
donations 22, 65, 96
Donnybrook *146*
Doric Order 104, *135–6*, 154, 156, 194–6
Dorset, duke of 34
Dorset Street 107
Down Survey 35–6, 183
drinking, illegal 123, 143, 187, 190
Drogheda, earl of 99
Drogheda Street 46–7
Dublin
    hospitals (*see* hospitals, Dublin)
    maps *140, 141*
        Monto *177, 178, 192*
        streets and hospitals *15, 17, 29, 45, 58, 62, 77, 146*
        Wide Streets Commissioners *108, 109*
    motto 174
    rural life in city **39–43**
Dublin Castle 96, 115
    British executive 95, 112, 144, 148, 168
Dublin Corporation 112
Dublin Evening Post 121, 141, 148
Dublin Journal 26–7, 59–60, 98–9, 100–1
Dublin Metropolitan Police 191

Dublin Society 38, 74
Duff, Frank 187, 190
Dunkin, Reverend William 34

Easter 1916 197
Elliot Place, Monto *188*
employment 72–3, 177
enclosure, parliamentary 37, 38
Encyclopaedia Britannica 177
enfilade system 41, 46
Ensor, John 46, 76, 77, 79, 153
entertainment. *see* Kildare House; music; New Pleasure Gardens; social life; theatre
Essay on Hospitals **82–6**
Essay on the Population of Dublin 182, 183
Exact Survey 27, 28, 29, 41, 43, 47, 54
examinations, medical 23
executions 117–18, 120
experimentation, medical 23–4, 29–33

façades, building **89–93**, 115, 121, 154, 156, 175, 194, 196, 197
    Assembly Rooms 111, 113–14
    Lying-in Hospital 44, 55, 56, 66, 67, 79, 136
    Newgate Gaol 116–17, **118–20**
Faithful Place, Monto *189*
Fane, John (Earl of Westmoreland) 128, 141, 148
farming and farmers 38, 199
'fatal tree,' Saint Stephen's Green 118
Faulkner's Journal 33, 59–60, 98–9, 100–1
fee, admission 50–1, 59
fever 88, 102, 158, 182
Fielding, Henry *quote* 41–2, 125–6
Filarette, Antonio 157
fire, Hôtel Dieu 158
fireworks 54
Fishamble Street Music Hall 33
FitzGerald, Emily (countess of Kildare) 34, *35*, 43, 133
FitzGerald, George 34
FitzGerald, James (earl of Kildare) 34, *35*
FitzGerald, Lord Edward 144
FitzGerald, Robert (earl of Kildare) 39
FitzGerald, Thomas Robert (second duke of Leinster) 128
Fitzwilliam, Lord 142
Fitzwilliam estate 109, 121
fluxing 165–6
Foster, Edward *Essay on Hospitals* **82–6**, 158
Foster, Francis *Thoughts for the Times but Chiefly on the Profligacy of Our Women* 32
Foster, John 111
Foucault, Michel 72–3, 86, 117, 131, 149, 157, 174
Foundling Hospital 16, *17*, 18, 19, 26, 115, 134, *165*
France, venereal disease in 146, 148, 161
Fraser, Murray 112, 197
Frederick Street, North 107, 111
Free Trade agreement 100
French revolution 142, 143, 144, 145, 174, 181, 182
French Street 178
funds and fundraising 22, 127. *see also under* Assembly Rooms; British Administration; Hospital for Incurables; Lying-in Hospital; Mosse Bartholomew; Westmoreland Lock Hospital
Galilei, Alessandro 37
gambling 143
Gandon, James 97, 110, 113, 159, 196
gaols **116–20**
gardens. *see* Cuper's Gardens; New Pleasure Gardens; Ranelagh Gardens; Vauxhall Gardens
    used for sexual pleasure **124–6**
Gardiner, Luke 46–7, 96–7, 108, 109, 111
Gardiner, Right Honorable Charles 79
gender separation 134–5, 165, 168, 184
General Post Office 193, 194, *196,* 197
General Treatise of Architecture in Five Books 135–6
General Valuation of Ireland 181–2
Gentleman and Citizen's Almanack 18, 22, 28, 65, 75, 150–1, 152
Gentlemen of Hughes's Club 98–9
George II, King 66
George's Lane 13, 27, *146,* 147
gonorrhoea 179
Gore, Sir Arthur (Lord Sudley) 66, 75
governors. *See under* Hospital for Incurables; Lying-in Hospital; Steeven's Hospital; Westmoreland Hospital
Grafton Street 178
Granby Row 77, 102
Grattan, Henry 113, 115
Great Britain Street 142

Handel's *Esther* 33
Handel's *Messiah* 34
Handel's *Music for the Royal Fireworks* 54
hangings 117–18, 120
Hardwicke Fever Hospital 159
Hazelwood House, County Sligo 39
Hemyng, Bracebridge 184
Hervey, Frederick Augustus (Lord Bristol) 128
Hibernia Curiosa 49–50
Hibernian Journal 54
Hibernian Magazine 48, 124
hierarchy, household **56–9**, 134
Higgins, Benjamin 25
Holister, William 55
Hospital for Incurables 16, *17, 90,* 94, **150–5**, 199
    architecture *90,* 153–4, *155,* 173
    funding 151
    governors 151
Hospital of King Charles 16
hospitals, Dublin
    in the eighteenth century **16–24** (*see also* Foundling Hospital; Hospital for Incurables; Lying-in Hospital; Mercer's Hospital; Royal Hospital Kilmainham; Saint Patrick's Hospital; Steeven's Hospital; voluntary hospitals; Westmoreland Lock Hospital)
    hospital practice in the eighteenth century 23–4
    location, construction and administration **82–9**
    old hospitals *versus* new hospitals **16–20**

Hôtel Dieu, Paris 20, 25, 129, 146, 158
House of Commons, Speaker 163
House of Correction 115
House of Industry 115, 154, 181
House of Lords, chambers extended 110–11
Howard, John 88, 120, 155
Hugo, Victor 185
Humbert, George 144
Hume, Sir Gustavus 39
hygiene 88

illness, terminal 173
Illustrious Order of Saint Patrick **95–103,** 113
improvement, ideologies of 73–4, 75
'incurable,' definition of 150–3
infanticide 26
inmates 90, 137–40, 175, 176, 200
Ionic Order *135–6,* 196
Ireland, militarised society (1790s) 144–5
Irish Builder 27, 152
Irish produce 100–1
Irish Society (ode) 180

James I (VI Scotland), King 36
James II, King 35
Jebb, Frederick 32
Jervis estate 39–40
Johnston, Francis
 other institutions designed by **174–6,** 199
 Westmoreland Lock Hospital 164–5, 166
Johnston, Richard 97, **155–62,** 164, 167, 173
Jones, Inigo 36
Joyce, James *Ulysses* 173, 186–7, 189
Juno Lucina, statue of 66, 75

Kildare 169
Kildare, countess of (Emily FitzGerald) 34
Kildare, earl of (James FitzGerald) 34, 66
Kildare, earl of (Richard FitzGerald) 39
Kildare House *15,* **39–43,** *57*
 comparison between Lying-in Hospital and **43–6**
Kildare Lock Hospital *172,* 173
Kilwarden, Lord 147
Knights of Saint Patrick **95–103,** 113

labour force 38, 72–3
'Lambeth Wells' 125
land, ownership and transfer of **35–9**
landlords 38. *see also* land, ownership of
landscapes of pleasure **46–56**
'large room.' *See* Rotunda
La Touche, David 97, 111, 126, 127–8, 139
laundry **166–7,** 170–1
Lawson, Reverend *quotes* 70–2, 87
Lazars Hill 150
Leeson, Mrs 199–200
 clients and memoirs of **126–9,** 141
Leeson's Wood Street brothel **126–9**
Legion of Mary 191
legislation 37, 82, 103, 104–5, 115, 123, 142, 169, 179–80
Leinster, duke of 75, 78–9
Leinster, duke of (William Robert Fitzgerald) 95, 96–7, 99, 128

Leinster House 34, 41, 83
Leix-Offaly plantation (1556) 35
leprosy 149–50
Le Roy, Jean-Baptiste 158
listening-post, Monto used as 192
Locke, John 36
Lock Hospital 21, 25, 29, 141, *146,* 147. *See also* Westmoreland Lock Hospital
Lock Penitentiary 137, 138, *141,* 142
Logan, William *The Great Social Evil* 173, 181, 184, 185, 186
London 79
London Hospital *89*
London Labour and the London Poor 184
Lord Bective's House 39
lottery ticket *56*
Lying-in Hospital 16, 22, **58–60,** 122, *125,* 199, 200. *see also* Assembly Rooms; New Pleasure Gardens; Rotunda
 admissions procedure **129–134,** 59, 145–6
 ambiguities and contradictions **129–34**
 architecture **27–9,** 43–6, *58, 60–1, 62, 64, 67, 74, 81, 100*
 changes after Mosse's death **75–7**
 chapel 60–1, *62,* **66–71,** 74, **134–7**
 comparison between Kildare House and 43–6
 debt 65, 75, 76
 entry to 59, *64,* 83
 founding of 13–14, 22, **24–7**
 funding and fundraising 14, 22, 60, 65, 76, 87, 102, 104
 governors 22, 34, 63, 65, 75–6, 99–100, 103, 104, 111, 121, 123, 134, 161
 layout **60–2,** *100*
 location and description of *15,* **27–9**
 management of children 73, 75
 mortality rates 81–2, 88, 131
 opening ceremony 61–3, 64–5, 81
 patients 64–5, 96, **129–34**
 records **25–7,** 53, 71, 81–2, 87–8, **129–34**
 visiting hours 59–60
McParland, Edward 107, 109, 111, 196
Magdalen Asylum **137–40,** 141, *170,* 199
Magee, John 121, 122, 141, 148
Malton, John 93–4, 104, 113
Man-Midwifery Dissected 30–1
Manners, Charles (duke of Rutland) 96, 113, *114,* 127
maps *140, 141*
Monto *177, 178, 192*
 streets and hospitals *15, 17, 29, 45, 58, 62, 77, 146*
 Wide Streets Commissioners *108, 109*
marital infidelities 128, 133, 184
Marlborough Bowling Green (1745) *47,* 48, 51, *52,* 54, 55, 124
masquerade 126, 127, 128
maternity hospitals **13–16, 24–7.** *see also* Lying-in Hospital; voluntary hospitals
 controversy **29–33**
Mayhew, Henry 169, 184, 185
Meath Hospital 21, 22

memoirs, Mrs Leeson's **126–9**
Mercer's Hospital 16, *17, 19,* 21, 25, 29, 33, 94
Merrion Square 109
middle-class 121, 138, 182
 interest in Monto 186, 187
 women and family values 184
midwifery, male 14, **24–7**
 controversy **29–33,** 129
 social implications 24
 training 104
Militant groups 38, 95, 144
military 144–5, 160, 169
 hospitals 160–1
 presence 167–8, 191–2
 and prostitution 143, 148, 177, 180–1
Miscellanea Medica (medical notebook) 31–2
Monasticum Hibernicum 94
Monto
 the creation of *177*–**82**
 labyrinth of vice **186–93,** 199
Mosse, Bartholomew 31, 38, 45–6, 54, 63, 71, 134
 background and career 16, 34–5
 commissions artists 66, 68
 death 68, **75–7**
 funding and fundraising 14, 33–4, 60, 65, 132
 and Lying-in Hospital 13–14, 25, 26, 28–9 (*see also* Lying-in Hospital; New Pleasure Gardens)
 nursing, clothing and maintenance scheme 73, 75
moralists 142–3, **169–71**
morality 142–3, **162–7,** 182–6
 management of **167–73**
 and prostitution **169–71,** 179–80
Mornington, earl of (Richard Wellesley) 99, 128
mortality rates 81–2, 88, 131
Mosse, Mrs 65
Mosse, Reverend Thomas 75, 87
motto, Dublin 174
Mountjoy Square 121, 182
Murray, T.A. 158
music 33, 34, 50, 53, 54, 79, 80

Naper, Esq. W. 43
National and Political Observations on the Bills of Mortality 183
national security, issues of 148, 160, 169
Naval Hospital, Stonehouse, England 160
Nelson, Lord 194–5
Nelson's Pillar 194–5, 197
Nesbitt, Dr Ezekial 75–6
Newgate Gaol, Dublin 116–17, *118–19, 174,* 175, 199
Newgate Gaol, London 117, *118–19,* 120
New Pleasure Gardens 43, 59, 77, *103,* 104, 122
 admission fee 50–1, 55–6, 58
 disorderly conduct 54–5, 123
 entertainment 13, 16, **49–51, 53–6,** 76, **78–80,** 121
 setting for sexual pleasure 124–6
 vice and closure **140–3**
 walls removed 103–4, 123–4
Nightingale, Florence 87
Nihell, Elizabeth *Treatise on the Art of Midwifery* 32

INDEX

Notes on Hospitals 87
Nugent-Temple-Grenville, Lord Lieutenant George 95
Oakboys 38
Obientia Civium Urbis Felicitus (Dublin City motto) 174
obstetricians. *see* Bartholomew Mosse; midwifery, male
O'Connell Street. *see* Sackville Street
ode 180
Orange, William of 35, 37, 95
orchestra 53, 79, 80
orphans 25–6
Ospedale Maggiore (plan) 157
Ould, Fielding 75, 76
outcasts. *See* disease; leprosy; prostitution
out-patients department 87
overcrowding, hospital 102

paintings 40, 93–4, 95, 104
Palace Row 77
Palladian architecture 89–90, 153–4
  big houses 36, 37, 39–46, 56–8, 77–8
  hospitals (*see* Hospital for Incurables; Lying-in Hospital; Westmoreland Lock Hospital)
  Lying-in chapel 66–71
  villa 36, 37, 39, 83, 86, 89, 90, 153–4
Palladio, Andrea 36
Parent-Duchâtelet, A.J.B. *De la Prostitution dans la Ville de Paris* 183–4, 185
Paris, prostitutes in 148–9, 183–4, 185
Parliament, dissolution of 145
Parliamentary funding 65, 75, 76, 79, 102, 111, 162, 168
Parliament Street 110, 113, 115, 116
patients 59, 64–5, 96
  admission 59, 129–34, 148, 156–7
  experimentation 23–4, **29–33**
  segregation of 90, 157–8, 160, 163–4, 165, 168
  venereal 155, 156, 157–8, 160–1, **162–7, 168–70,** 173
patrons 14–16, 22, 65–6, 73–4, 75–6, 101
pavilion plan 89, 111, **157–60,** 163, 173
peasants 38, 40, 199
Penal Laws 22
pensioners 50
Percival, Dr 159
Petty, Sir William *Down Survey* 35–6, 183
Philip, Ambrose 33
piano nobile (first floor) 57–8, 61, 66, 83, 89
pilgrims 150
plantation, Protestant 35
pleasure, landscapes of **46–56**
Pleasure Gardens. *See* New Pleasure Gardens
Plunkett, Peg (Mrs Leeson) 126–9
Police Act of 1786 104–5
Poor House 16, *19,* 26
population growth and density 38, 47, 199
Porter, Mrs 128
porticos 110–11, 116, 194, 196
poverty 63, 115, 120–1, 181–2, 188–9, 190, 197

Powerscourt House, County Wicklow 39
pregnancy and delivery 24–5, 31–2, 81–2, 128–9
Priory of the Knights Hospitallers 94
prisons **116–20**
productivity and Protestantism 65–74
professional class 16, 22, 24–5, 121
Promenade d'un Français en Irlande 126
prosecution, threats of 123
prostitution 121, 122, 133, **140–3,** 199–200
  decline in arrests 179, 180
  high-class **126–9,** 133
  intervention and surveillance of 124, **145–50,** 183
  lower-class 121, 140, 141, 143, 181, 185, 193, 197
  in Monto **177–82, 186–93**
  Mrs Leeson's clients and memoirs **126–9**
  in Paris 148–9, 183
  surveys and studies 182, 183–6
  upper-class 188
  venereal disease and **168–71,** 173
Prostitution: Considered in its Moral, Social and Sanitary Aspects 184
Protestantism 16, 22, 26, 35, 37–8, 65–6. *See also* Anglo-Irish
  land-owners **35–9**
  militia 95, 144
  and productivity **65–74**
  values 72–3, 74
public holidays 60
publicity 54, 56, 101
public spaces 104, 106, **182–6, 188–90,** 200. *See also* New Pleasure Gardens; social spaces; urban spaces
puerperal fever 88, 102
purpose-built hospitals 13–14, 21, 89

Queenstown 169

Rainsford Street *146,* 147
Ranelagh Gardens, Dublin 51, 55
Ranelagh Gardens, London 50, *51,* 79, 126
1798 rebellion 142, 143, 144, 145, 174, 181, 182
records, hospital 23, **25–7,** 53, 71, 81–2, 87–8, **129–34,** 200
recruitment, British 144
red-light district 122, 193. *see also* brothels; Monto; prostitution
'red whore' 185, 192–3
rehabilitation 170–1
residents, Rutland Square **103–6**
retirement homes. *See* Chelsea Hospital; Royal Hospital Kilmainham
Richmond House of Correction 174, 175, 191, 195
Richmond Lunatic Asylum 174
Richmond Penitentiary 174, *175,* 176
Richmond Surgical 173
Ridotto al Fresco 126
Robinson, William 93
Rock, Dr 97
Rocque, John
  Exact Survey 27, 28, 29, 41, 43, 47, 54
  Rocque's Plan 107, 108

Ross, Sir John Foster (Lieutenant Colonel) 193
Rotunda, Ranelagh, London 79, *80*
Rotunda Hospital 76, 96, *100,* 122, *125,* 142, 143, 194. *See also* Assembly Rooms; Lying-in Hospital
  arrival of **78–82**
  report 97–8
Royal Barracks 178
Royal Charter 34
Royal College of Physicians 34
Royal Exchange 110, 112–13, *114, 115–16, 117*
Royal Hospital, Kilmainham 16, *17, 19, 20, 46, 92, 93–4,* 159
Royal Hospital, London *51*
Royal Irish Academy 94
Royal Military Infirmary *92,* 93, 159–60
rural life in Dublin city **39–43**
Rutland, duke of (Charles Manners) 96, 127
  coat of arms 113, *114*
Rutland Square **103–6,** *141,* 182
  paving and lighting of 103–4, 123

Sackville, Lionel 47
Sackville Mall 47, 48–9, 50, 106, 108, 109, 110
Sackville Street 47, 48–9, 106–7, *108, 109*–10, 111, 121, 182, **194–8**
Sackville Street, Lower 121
St George's Church 194
St James's Hospital 94, 150
St James's Square, (20), London 40
St John's Hospital 94
St Lazare Hospital, France 148, 149
St Patrick 95, 101
St Patrick's Cathedral 95
St Patrick's Day parade 95–6
St Patrick's Hospital 21, 25, 29, 65, 90–1, 115, 153, 161
St Stephen's Green 47, 48, 51, 55, *140,* 178
St Stephen's Hospital 94
St Thomas's Hospital, London 146–7
sanitary inspection 148
Santiago de Compostella 150
Scamozzi, Vincenzo 135
sculptures 66, 75
sedan chairs tax 104, 105
segregation
  gender 134–5, 165, 168, 184
  patients 90, 157–8, 160, 163–4, 165, 168
  public spaces 134–5, 184
Semple, George 90, 153
Semple, John 45
Serlio, Sebastiano 110, 194
servants 57, 58, 59
sexual harassment 32
sexual pleasures and behaviour **124–9,** 133, **140–3,** 179. *See also* prostitution
Shannon, Lord 66, 75, 99
Shaw's directory 181–2
Sheriff's Prison 120
Smock Alley Theatre 33
Smyth, William 137
social class 14, 134
  separation and proximity 63, 134–5, **137–40,** 188

social life 47–9, **50–6**, 79–80. *See also* Kildare House; music; New Pleasure Gardens; theatre
social reformers 186, 187, 190, 191
social spaces **47–51**, 106, 110, **182–6**. *See also* New Pleasure Gardens; public spaces; urban spaces
Society for Suppression of Vice 185
Soldiers' Infirmary 115
sponsors 14–16, 22, 65–6, 73–4, 75–6, 101
State of the Hospital (report) 25–6
statisticians and reports 18, 26–7, **181–6**
statutes 66, 75
Steeven's Hospital 16, *17, 21,* 25, 29, 46, *92,* 93, 115, 145, 150, 173
  governors 161–2
Stevenson, Robert 43
Steyne Hospital 150
Stone, George (archbishop of Armagh) 34
streets, widening of 46–7, **106–14, 115–22**
streetwalkers 121, 140, 141, 178, 185, 193
Sudley, Lord (Sir Arthur Gore) 66, 75
surgeons 20, 22–3
  relationship with patients 23
  voluntary hospitals and 20, 22–3
surveillance, disciplinary 104, 124, 148–9, **174–6**, 185
surveys 27, 28, 29, 35–6
  poor and prostitution **182–6**
syphilis 165–6, 179

Taafe, Denis 120
'Taste-à-la-mode 1745' *47,* 48, 124
'Taste-à-la-mode, 1790' 124–5
taxation 103–4, 105
Taylour, Thomas (earl of Bective) 128
Temple Bar 115
'Temple of Flora' 125
tenements 181–2, 188–90
theatre 33–4, 48
  model for urban design 110, 112
  tragic theatre set *195*
Theatre Royal, Crow Street *48*
The Distressed Mother 33–4
The Great Social Evil 173, 184
The New Booth 33
Thom's directory 181
Thoughts for the Times but Chiefly on the Profligacy of Our Women 32
tourism 200
Townsend, Viscount 150
Townsend Street *146,* 147, 150, 161

Treatise on Civil Architecture 78
Treatise on the Art of Midwifery 32
Treatise on the Management of Pregnant and Lying-in Women 88
Trench, Frederick 96, 97, 102–3, 104, 111, 113, 142
trials, clinical 161
Trinity College 39, 46, 107
Tyrone, earl of 99
Tyrone House *15,* 39, 40

Ulysses 173, 186–7
unemployment 38, 177
United Irishmen 144
upper class 47, 48, 199
  midwifery 24–5
  sexual pleasures **124–9**, 133
  social interaction with other classes **124–9**, 134–5, 137, 188
urban spaces 110, 194, 197–8, 199. *See also* New Pleasure Gardens; public spaces; social spaces
utilitarian hospital, Foster's **82–6**

Vance, Surgeon 129
Van Nost, John 66, 75
Vauxhall Gardens, London 49–50, 51, 59, 79, 124, 125, 126
venereal disease 64, 128–9, 141, **145–50**, 155, 161, 163–5, 179
  females and **167–73**
ventilation, ideas on **82–8, 158–60,** 165
Vierpyl, Simon 53, 79
View of Dublin (painting) 93–4
Violante, Madame 33
Vitruvius, Marcus 110, 194
  De Architectura 135
Vitruvius Britannica 38
voluntary hospitals **14–20**, 94, 147, 150
  founded **20–2**
Volunteers 95, 96

Wales, prince of 14, 66
Walker, Reverend John 137
Walpole, Horace 79
war 144, 174, 180, 181, 192. *See also* 1798 rebellion
Warburton, Whitelaw and Walsh 112–13, 138, 145, 152, 154, 162, 165–6, 194, 196
wards 73–4, 129, 154, 155, **155–60,** 164, 165–6. *see also* pavilion plan
War of Independence 192
Warren, Nathaniel (Lord Mayor of Dublin) 128
waterfall 53

Watson's *Almanack* 18, 22, 28, 65, 75, 150–1, 152
wealth 38, 56–7, 190
Weber, Max 72
Wellesley, Richard (earl of Mornington) 128
West, Robert 67
Westmoreland, earl of (John Fane) 128, 141, 148
Westmoreland Lock Hospital **145–50,** 199, 200. *See also* Lock Hospital
  admissions procedure 163–4
  architecture **155–60, 162–7,** *171*
  extensions **155–67**
  funding 162, 168
  governors 161, 163, 164, 167–8
  laundry 166–7, 170–1
  moral management **167–73**
  patients 148, 155, 156–8, 160, 163–4, 165–6, 168
  staffing problems 163
Westmoreland Street 107, 108, 111, 194
Wheatley, Francis 95
Whig administration 36, 37
White, Charles *Treatise on the Management of Pregnant and Lying-in Women* 88
Whiteboys 38
White Cross Vigilance Association 179
Whitelaw, James *An Essay on the Population of Dublin* 182, 183
Whitworth, earl of 196
Wide Streets Commissioners **106–14, 115–22**
Wilde, Sir William 27, 131–2, 183
Wilkins, William 194
Wilson, Richard 40
Wolfe, Arthur 147
Wolfe Tone, Theobald 142
Wollstonecraft, Mary 23
women 199–200. *See also* Magdalen asylum; prostitution; venereal disease
  childbirth **24–7,** 31–2, 63, 81–2
  deaths 26, 131
  lower class 184, 199
  middle-class 184
  midwifery and 24–5, 71
  working class 73, 184, 190. *See also* poverty; prostitution
Wotton, Sir Henry 135
Wynn, Sir Watkin Williams 40

Young, Arthur 110